Essential Questions in Paediatrics for MRCPCH – Volume 1

Edited by

Dr R M Beattie BSc MBBS MRCP FRCPCH
Consultant Paediatric Gastroenterologist
Paediatric Medical Unit
Southampton General Hospital
Southampton

and

Dr M P Champion BSc MBBS MRCP MRCPCH
Consultant in Paediatric Metabolic Medicine
Evelina Children's Hospital
Guy's and St. Thomas' Hospital NHS Trust
London

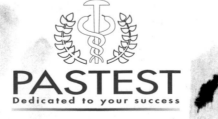

PASTEST
Dedicated to your success

First edition 2004

618 92   BEA

ISBN: 1 901198 99 5

A catalogue record for this book is available from the British Library.

The information contained within this book was obtained by the authors from
reliable sources. However, while every effort has been made to ensure its
accuracy, no responsibility for loss, damage or injury occasioned to any person
acting or refraining from action as a result of information contained herein can
be accepted by the publisher or the authors.

PasTest Revision Books and Intensive Courses

*PasTest has been established in the field of postgraduate medical education
since 1972, providing revision books and intensive study courses for doctors
preparing for their professional examinations. Books and courses are available
for the following specialties:*

MRCP Part 1 and Part 2, MRCPCH Part 1 and Part 2, MRCOG, DRCOG, MRCGP,
MRCPsych, DCH, FRCA, MRCS and PLAB.

For further details contact:

PasTest Ltd, Freepost, Knutsford, Cheshire, WA16 7BR
Tel: 01565 752000   Fax: 01565 650264
Email: enquiries@pastest.co.uk   Web site: www.pastest.co.uk

Typeset by Saxon Graphics Ltd, Derby
Printed by MPG Ltd, Bodmin, Cornwall

Contents

Contributors List

Dr R M Beattie BSc MBBS MRCP FRCPCH
Consultant Paediatric Gastroenterologist
Paediatric Medical Unit
Southampton General Hospital
Southampton

Michael L Capra MBBCh DCH Dip.Obst MRCP MMedSci (Clinical education)
Assistant Professor
Division of Haematology/Oncology
The Hospital for Sick Children
Toronto
Canada

Mike Champion BSc MBBS MRCP MRCPCH
Consultant in Paediatric Metabolic Medicine
Evelina Children's Hospital
Guy's and St. Thomas' Hospital NHS Trust
London

Helen M Goodyear MBChB MRCP FRCPCH MD MMEd
Consultant Paediatrician and Associate Postgraduate Dean
Department of Child Health
Birmingham Heartlands Hospital
Bordesley Green East
Birmingham

Heather Mitchell BM.BCh MA MRCP MRCPCH MRCGP DCH DRCOG
SpR in Paediatric Endocrinology
Department of Paediatric Endocrinology
University College London Hospitals
London

Joanne Philpot BA MBBS MD MRCPCH
Consultant Paediatrician
Paediatric Department
Wexam Park Hospital
Slough

Waseem Qasim BMedSci MRCP MRCPCH, PhD
Molecular Immunology
Institute of Child Health
London

Fiona M Regan MBChB MRCPCH
Paediatric Endocrine Clinical Research Fellow
University of Cambridge
Department of Paediatrics
Addenbrooke's Hospital
Cambridge

Stephen Tomlin BPharm MRPharmS AFNPP (CPP)
Principal Paediatric Pharmacist
Pharmacy Department
Guy's and St Thomas' Hospital NHS Trust
London

Robert M R Tulloh BM BCh MA DM MRCP (Paeds) FRCPCH
Consultant Paediatric Cardiologist
Department of Congenital Disease
Guy's and St Thomas' Hospital NHS Trust
London

Mr R A Wheeler MS FRCS LLB (Hons) FRCPCH
Consultant Paediatric and Neonatal Surgeon
Southampton General Hospital
Southampton

Louise C Wilson BSc MBChB FRCP
Consultant in Clinical Genetics
Institute of Child Health
Department of Genetics
London

Introduction

These revision texts have been written to accompany Essential Revision Notes in Paediatrics for the MRCPCH but are also relevant for part one of the DCH examination. The questions, in the new format are designed to help facilitate revision for the MRCPCH part one examination. The books are split by subject to aid revision planning. Each question has a detailed explanation and so the text can be used as a stand alone revision aid.

The candidate is advised to consult the RCPCH website for up to date information regarding the exam. The information below is taken from the website and is correct at the time of going to press.

The MRCPCH Part One examination consists of two papers.

Paper One A (Basic Child Health) will focus on the areas of child health that are relevant to those who will be working with children in their medical careers, not just those entering mainstream hospital-based paediatrics. The areas to be tested will be those conditions likely to be seen in 6 to 12 months of hospital, community or primary care practice.

Paper One B (Extended Paediatrics) will focus on the more complex paediatric problem-solving skills not tested in Paper One A, and on the scientific knowledge underpinning paediatrics. This is equivalent to the current MRCPCH Part One paper.

Candidates for MRCPCH must successfully complete both Paper One A and One B before being allowed to enter MRCPCH Part Two. .

Paper One A (Basic Child Health) will replace the current Diploma in Child Health (DCH) written papers.

The papers will consist of

Multiple true-false questions used to test knowledge when there is an absolute Yes/No answer.

Best of Five questions used to test judgement and experience. A simple statement or short clinical scenario leads into five options. All could be possible but only one is completely or the most correct. The candidate has to choose the best option.

Extended matching questions (EMQs) are used in the same way as Best of Five questions. In this case a list of 10 possible answers is offered with three statements or clinical scenarios. The candidate chooses the best option from the introductory list. Again, all could be possible but only one is completely or the most correct.

Further details on the make up of the three types of questions are on the college website. There are also downloadable sample papers which should be reviewed.

We are indebted in the production of this book to the many authors who have enthusiastically contributed chapters and to Kirsten Baxter at Pastest for her enthusiasm and expertise in helping pull the book together.

Mark Beattie

Mike Champion

June 2004

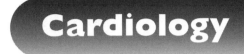

Cardiology

Robert Tulloh

Multiple Choice Questions

1. On the first day of life the following may be found in neonates with congenital heart disease

- ○ A a harsh pan-systolic murmur with the diagnosis of ventricular septal defect
- ○ B severe cyanosis in unobstructed total anomalous pulmonary venous connection
- ○ C a harsh systolic murmur in transposition of the great arteries without associated defect
- ○ D severe acidosis and poor pulses with hypoplastic left heart syndrome
- ○ E severe cyanosis and acidosis in a baby with Down syndrome and atrioventricular septal defect

2. The following are risk factors in fetal life for congenital heart disease

- ○ A Down syndrome
- ○ B increased thickness of nuchal translucency on 20-week fetal anomaly scan
- ○ C maternal phenylketonuria
- ○ D echodensities in the left ventricle on fetal ultrasound
- ○ E maternal epilepsy controlled with phenytoin

3. The following is true of persistent arterial duct

- ○ A it is defined as persistence of ductal patency beyond 1 week after the date the baby should have been born
- ○ B on auscultation, a continuous murmur in the right infraclavicular area is heard
- ○ C it may present as heart failure with poor peripheral pulses
- ○ D closure is usually undertaken in catheter laboratory with coil or device at 1 year
- ○ E if large, surgical ligation is recommended at 1–3 months

questions

4. The following statements about transposition of the great arteries are true

○ A there is an association with coarctation of the aorta
○ B arterial switch is operation of choice, undertaken before 2 weeks
○ C the condition is detected antenatally in 50% of cases
○ D presentation can occur upon closure of the arterial duct
○ E the arrangement of the coronary arteries is a major factor in determining the success of the surgical repair

5. The following is true of Eisenmenger syndrome

○ A affected children are typically teenagers
○ B it can be seen in children with Down syndrome
○ C it is usually secondary to an untreated ventricular septal defect or atrioventricular septal defect
○ D the pulmonary component of the second heart sound is quiet on auscultation
○ E the electrocardiogram shows left ventricular hypertrophy

6. The following statements about hypoplastic left heart syndrome are true

○ A prostaglandin E is not required pre-operatively
○ B operation is usually undertaken at 3–5 days of life
○ C if sick, the infants present with absent brachial and femoral pulses
○ D can be indistinguishable clinically from critical aortic stenosis
○ E 30% have associated coarctation of the aorta

7. Regarding totally anomalous pulmonary venous connections (TAPVC)

○ A there is usually no dysmorphic syndrome associated with the condition
○ B supra-cardiac TAPVC to the innominate vein is the commonest form to occur
○ C infra-cardiac TAPVC can become obstructed at the level of the diaphragm
○ D TAPVC is a duct-dependent lesion
○ E it is never found with right atrial isomerism

8. A Blalock–Taussig shunt is the treatment of choice for

○ A tetralogy of Fallot with pulmonary atresia in the newborn period
○ B tricuspid atresia with pulmonary atresia
○ C ventricular septal defect and coarctation of the aorta
○ D interruption of the aortic arch
○ E hypoplastic left heart syndrome

9. The following associations are correctly paired

- ○ A totally anomalous pulmonary venous connections and right atrial isomerism
- ○ B two morphologic right lungs and right atrial isomerism
- ○ C left-sided liver and right atrial isomerism
- ○ D asplenia and left atrial isomerism
- ○ E malrotation of the small bowel and left atrial isomerism

10. Characteristic cardiac features of William syndrome include

- ○ A subvalvar aortic stenosis
- ○ B peripheral pulmonary artery stenosis
- ○ C transposition of the great arteries
- ○ D atrial septal defect
- ○ E hypoplastic pulmonary arteries

11. Children with Di George syndrome

- ○ A have 21q11.2 deletion
- ○ B can have a normally functioning thymus gland
- ○ C have high plasma calcium levels
- ○ D often have palate abnormalities
- ○ E require irradiated blood to prevent graft-versus-host disease, if they are T cell-deficient

12. The following statements about Kawasaki disease are true

- ○ A not usually associated with dysmorphic syndrome
- ○ B it is associated with bilateral purulent conjunctivitis
- ○ C high dose steroid therapy is the treatment of choice
- ○ D 40% of affected children develop coronary artery aneurysms without treatment
- ○ E aspirin should not be used due to risk of Reye syndrome

13. The following is true of dilated cardiomyopathy

- ○ A it can be associated with vitamin D deficiency
- ○ B the most common cause is post viral infection
- ○ C anomalous coronary artery should be excluded using echocardiography
- ○ D there may be a family history of sudden unexplained death
- ○ E it may be associated with mitochondrial disease

14. Causes of long Q–T interval include

- ○ A Romano–Ward syndrome
- ○ B Jervell–Lange–Nielsen syndrome
- ○ C hypercalcaemia
- ○ D hypomagnesaemia
- ○ E hyperthermia

15. Congenital heart block diagnosed in fetal life

- ○ A may be associated with structural heart disease
- ○ B has a poor prognosis if there is hydrops in utero
- ○ C should be paced immediately after birth if the heart rate is below 60 beats per minute
- ○ D is due to maternal systemic lupus erythematosus (SLE) in 70% of cases
- ○ E can be treated with neonatal isoprenaline

16. The following is true of tetralogy of Fallot

- ○ A It often presents with a loud harsh murmur at the upper sternal edge on day 1
- ○ B murmur is due to the presence of a ventricular septal defect
- ○ C the Rastelli operation should be performed to correct Fallot at 1 year of age
- ○ D if severely cyanosed at birth, a Blalock–Taussig shunt is the best management option
- ○ E right bundle branch block often occurs after surgical correction

17. The following statements about pulmonary stenosis are true

- ○ A critical pulmonary stenosis causes cyanosis
- ○ B the right ventricle may be small
- ○ C pulmonary stenosis is frequently associated with coronary artery fistulae
- ○ D 80% of those who undergo balloon dilatation will require no further treatment
- ○ E less than 10% will require surgery in the form of a trans-annular patch

18. Coarctation of the aorta

- ○ A subclavian flap is the commonest surgical repair
- ○ B usually presents with systemic hypertension and radiofemoral delay
- ○ C is associated with Noonan syndrome
- ○ D repair is usually performed via a left lateral thoracotomy incision
- ○ E in 50% there is a bicuspid aortic valve

19. Innocent murmurs

○ A are always due to normal flow around the heart – never to cardiac pathology

○ B may resolve on lying down, compared with sitting up

○ C can be soft diastolic murmurs at the left sternal edge

○ D children with innocent murmurs should have antibiotic prophylaxis prior to dental procedures

○ E are more likely to lead to congenital heart disease in offspring

20. Characteristic cardiac features of Noonan syndrome include

○ A hypertrophic cardiomyopathy

○ B coarctation of the aorta

○ C pulmonary valve stenosis

○ D ventricular septal defect

○ E pulmonary hypertension

Best of Five Questions

21. **A 1-month-old baby presents to A&E with breathlessness and poor feeding. Her mother says she has been getting worse over the last week. On examination she is found to have a large liver, a respiratory rate of 60/min, and an active precordium with a soft murmur. Her oxygen saturations are 94% and she has good femoral pulses. What would you advise as the MOST appropriate treatment?**

   ○ A Start digoxin and diuretics and see in the clinic in 3 months time
   ○ B Start captopril in casualty and see in the clinic in 1 month
   ○ C Refer for immediate cardiac surgery
   ○ D Restrict milk feeds and fluids
   ○ E Start diuretics and admit to the ward for observation

22. **A 1-day-old baby who is otherwise asymptomatic presents with a loud harsh heart murmur at the left sternal edge. There are no features of heart failure present, the oxygen saturations are normal, and the electrocardiogram performed by the resident senior house officer is reported to be normal. What is the MOST likely diagnosis in this case?**

   ○ A Atrial septal defect
   ○ B Small muscular ventricular septal defect
   ○ C Large muscular ventricular septal defect
   ○ D Pulmonary stenosis
   ○ E Persistent arterial duct

23. **A new born, severely cyanosed baby is diagnosed as having tetralogy of Fallot following an echocardiogram performed on the ward. The baby is stabilised on intravenous medication, and the parents ask you to tell them what will happen next. You tell them the OPTIMAL management of the situation is to do which of the following?**

   ○ A The baby should be taken to theatre to have the ventricular septal defect closed
   ○ B The baby should be taken to theatre to have a Blalock–Taussig shunt inserted
   ○ C The baby should be taken to theatre to have a pulmonary artery band applied
   ○ D A balloon atrial septostomy is the treatment of choice to help reduce the cyanosis
   ○ E Giving high flow oxygen is enough for the time being and a corrective operation will be scheduled when the baby is 1-month-old

24. **A newborn baby presents cyanosed and unwell with a heart murmur at the left sternal edge. The chest radiograph shows massive cardiomegaly with a dilated right atrium and reduced pulmonary vascular markings. You are informed that the baby's mother has a history of bipolar depression and that she had been taking lithium during pregnancy. What is the MOST likely diagnosis?**

○ A Transposition of the great arteries
○ B Tetralogy of Fallot
○ C Tricuspid atresia
○ D Ebstein anomaly
○ E Pulmonary atresia, ventricular septal defect and collaterals

25. **You are asked to examine an 8-year-old child during an out-patient clinic. You notice a left lateral thoracotomy scar and detect a weak left brachial pulse. All other pulses are normal. There are no heart murmurs and the child is not cyanosed. What is your MOST likely conclusion?**

○ A Subclavian flap repair for coarctation of the aorta
○ B End-to-end anastomosis repair for coarctation of the aorta
○ C A pulmonary artery band operation has been performed
○ D A Blalock–Taussig shunt operation has been performed with a graft of the left subclavian artery forming the shunt
○ E Previous arterial duct ligation had been performed and the child now has a thrombotic occlusion of the left subclavian artery

· 26. **A 2-year-old boy presents with a murmur heard in both systole and diastole at the upper sternal edge, which disappears upon lying down. Physical examination was otherwise normal. He is a well, asymptomatic child and there are no signs of cardiac failure. You are told that his second cousin had a small ventricular septal defect, which closed spontaneously, and that his uncle had a heart attack aged 45. What do you consider to be the BEST management plan?**

○ A Refer for echocardiography and specialist opinion from a consultant paediatric cardiologist
○ B Perform an electrocardiogram, chest radiograph, and oxygen saturations and then refer for echocardiography
○ C Refer for genetic counselling and possible gene mapping studies
○ D Reassure them that the murmur is innocent
○ E Say that you suspect the murmur is caused by a persistent arterial duct, which should be coil-occluded to avoid the development of heart failure in the future

27. You are asked to review a 4-month-old girl in clinic. Her electrocardiogram shows a short P–R interval and giant QRS complexes. Echocardiography reveals evidence of hypertrophic cardiomyopathy. What is the most likely diagnosis?

○ A Pompe disease
○ B Lown–Ganong–Levine syndrome
○ C Hurler syndrome
○ D Noonan syndrome
○ E Wolf–Parkinson–White syndrome

Extended Matching Questions

28. Theme: Incidence of congenital heart disease

A   1 in 100
B   1 in 500
C   1 in 1000
D   1 in 10,000
E   1 in 100,000
F   1 in 1000,000
G   1 in 5000,000
H   1 in 10,000,000

In children with the disorders described below, which of the incidence rates listed above is nearest to the true incidence? Each option may be used once, more than once, or not at all.

○ 1. Hypoplastic left heart syndrome.
○ 2. Congenital heart disease.
○ 3. Ventricular septal defect.

29. Theme: Presentations of congenital heart disease

A   Atrial septal defect
B   Restrictive ventricular septal defect
C   Large apical muscular ventricular septal defect
D   Hypoplastic left heart syndrome
E   Partial anomalous pulmonary venous connection
F   Pulmonary stenosis
G   Transposition of the great arteries
H   Tetralogy of Fallot
I   Complete atrioventricular septal defect

Choose the option from those listed above which is most likely to result in the three scenarios described below. Each option may be used once, more than once, or not at all.

○ 1. A 2-day-old baby presents with breathlessness and poor feeding. On examination, she has a soft murmur with single second sound, a 4-cm liver, and her oxygen saturations are 65%.
○ 2. A collapsed 2-day-old baby presents on the postnatal ward, grey with absent pulses, no murmur, a 4-cm liver edge, and severe acidosis on a blood gas.
○ 3. At the pre-school check for 4-year-olds, a GP notices that a child is well, with no symptoms, and good exercise tolerance. There is a moderate ejection systolic heart murmur grade 3/6 at the upper left sternal edge with a fixed split second sound. The chest radiograph shows cardiomegaly, and electrocardiogram shows partial right bundle branch block and right ventricular hypertrophy.

questions

30. Theme: Dysrhythmias

A   Ice pack on the face
B   Valsalva manoeuvre
C   Intravenous adenosine
D   Synchronised DC cardioversion
E   Intravenous amiodarone
F   Defibrillation
G   Radiofrequency ablation
H   Sotalol
I   Oral digoxin

Choose the best treatment from those listed above for the following scenarios. Each option may be used once, more than once, or not at all.

○ 1. A 3-month-old presenting with narrow complex tachycardia at 300 beats/min.

○ 2. An unconscious 4-year-old found drowned in a pond, with ventricular fibrillation.

○ 3. Recurrent episodes of supraventricular tachycardia in a 7-year-old, despite prophylaxis.

answers

1. Congenital heart disease on the first day of life

Answers: D E

Babies presenting with left-to-right shunt will have no murmur or symptoms on the first day of life, since the pulmonary vascular resistance has yet to fall. Similarly, any common mixing disease, such as atrioventricular septal defect, can present with severe cyanosis on the first day of life with high pulmonary vascular resistance, before breathlessness and heart failure develop at 1 week of age or more. All the obstructed left heart lesions, such as coarctation of the aorta and hypoplastic left heart syndrome, tend to present with acidosis and weak pulses in the first few days of life.

2. Fetal risk factors for congenital heart disease

Answers: A B C E

The aetiology of congenital heart disease is largely multifactorial. Factors include inheritance, chromosomal abnormalities, and environmental factors. Drugs, such as alcohol or amphetamines, are associated with transposition of the great arteries, ventricular septal defects, and persistent arterial duct. Phenytoin is associated with pulmonary stenosis, aortic stenosis, coarctation of the aorta, or persistent arterial duct. Lithium is associated with Ebstein abnormality of the tricuspid valve, infections (particularly rubella, cytomegalovirus and other herpes viruses), maternal illnesses (eg diabetes mellitus leading to neonatal hypertrophic cardiomyopathy and systemic lupus erythematosus (anti-Ro and anti-La antibodies) increasing the risk of fetal complete heart block).

3. Persistent arterial duct

Answers: D E

There is abnormal persistence of the arterial duct beyond 1 month after the date the baby should have been born. Those children affected are usually asymptomatic and rarely develop heart failure. On auscultation, a continuous 'machinery' or systolic murmur at the left infraclavicular area is heard. The murmur is initially systolic but as the pulmonary vascular resistance falls, it becomes continuous in nature because there is a continual run-off of blood from the aorta to the pulmonary artery (as the pressure in the aorta is greater than the pulmonary artery throughout the cardiac cycle). Other clinical features include bounding pulses and wide pulse pressure. If the duct is large, chest radiography can demonstrate cardiomegaly and pulmonary plethora. Management is usually by closure in the cardiac catheter lab with a coil or device at 1 year of age. If large, surgical ligation may be undertaken aged 1–3 months. The presence of an arterial duct in a preterm baby is not congenital heart disease but these children have a higher incidence of persistent arterial duct.

4. Transposition of the great arteries

Answers: A B D E

In this condition, the aorta usually arises anteriorly from the right ventricle and the pulmonary artery arises posteriorly from the left ventricle. Deoxygenated blood is therefore returned to the body whilst oxygenated blood goes back to the lungs. If these two parallel circuits were completely separate, the condition would be incompatible with life. These children have high pulmonary blood flow and will be very cyanosed, unless there is an atrial septal defect, an arterial duct or ventricular septal defect, allowing mixing of the two circulations. Babies become cyanosed when the duct closes, thus reducing the mixing between the systemic and pulmonary circulations, but there is usually no murmur. Transposition of the great arteries may be associated with ventricular septal defect, coarctation of the aorta, or pulmonary stenosis. Management is to resuscitate the baby, followed by a balloon atrial septostomy at a cardiac centre in about 20% of cases (preferably via the umbilical vein). In the sick cyanosed newborn baby, a continuous intravenous infusion of prostaglandin E_1 or E_2 should be commenced to keep the duct open. Definitive repair in the form of the arterial switch operation will usually be undertaken before the baby is 2 weeks of age.

5. Eisenmenger syndrome

Answers: A B C

The Eisenmenger syndrome was first described in 1897 and occurs secondary to a large left-to-right shunt (usually a ventricular septal defect or atrioventricular septal defect) where the pulmonary hypertension leads to pulmonary vascular disease (increased resistance over many years). Eventually the flow through the defect is reversed (right-to-left) so the child becomes blue, typically at 10–15 years of age. There is not usually a significant heart murmur. Eventually, they develop right heart failure. Electrocardiogram shows right ventricular hypertrophy and strain pattern, with peaked P waves indicating right atrial hypertrophy. Management is largely supportive, as surgical closure is not possible when there is a right-to-left shunt. Diuretic and anticoagulant therapy may be required.

6. Hypoplastic left heart syndrome

Answers: B C D

Hypoplastic left heart syndrome is classically characterised by a right-ventricle-dependent systemic and pulmonary circulation associated with varying degrees of under-development of the left-sided cardiac structures. The mainstay of management of this condition in the UK is staged palliative reconstructive surgery. The first stage is the Norwood procedure, which is performed in the neonatal period and which enables the right ventricle to act as the systemic pump, and also allows blood to flow to the lungs via a systemic-to-pulmonary artery shunt. It is a common diagnosis (200–400 born annually in UK) and is usually diagnosed antenatally. A sick baby can present with absent femoral and brachial pulses but no murmur. Signs of right heart failure (large liver, low cardiac output) should be looked for; the child may also be breathless and severely acidotic. Management is to resuscitate and to commence prostaglandin E_1 or E_2 (5–20 ng/kg/min) followed by surgery (Norwood operation 3–5 days later). The next operation, a modified Glenn or Hemi-Fontan, is usually undertaken at 4–8 months of age, and the Fontan at about 3 years of age.

7. Totally anomalous pulmonary venous connections (TAPVC)

Answers: A B C

TAPVC occurs when the pulmonary veins have not made the normal connection to the left atrium during embryologic development. It is an uncommon diagnosis. The anatomical sites of anomalous venous drainage are divided into supra-cardiac (usually draining up to the innominate vein), intra-cardiac (draining into the right atrium or coronary sinus) and infra-cardiac (draining into the inferior vena cava or hepatic portal vein). If the veins become obstructed, they present on day 1–7 with cyanosis, respiratory difficulty and collapse, but usually no murmur. Signs of right heart failure should be checked for and the child may be breathless and severely acidotic. Affected children may present later up to any age if unobstructed, with a murmur or heart failure and failure to thrive, or even an incidental finding. Management of sick infants is to resuscitate and ventilate early, undergoing emergency surgery if obstructed. Prostaglandin is not effective because it is not a duct-dependent lesion.

8. Blalock–Taussig shunt

Answers: A B

Blalock–Taussig shunt is a tube of Gore-Tex, which connects the systemic circulation (usually either the subclavian artery or the innominate artery) with the pulmonary circulation (either the right or left branch of the pulmonary artery). It is put in place in order to ensure a secure low-pressure flow of blood to the lungs and thereby reduce cyanosis. Definitive repair of the underlying cardiac defect will be performed usually by age 18 months. In hypoplastic left heart syndrome a shunt is only part of the Norwood operation.

answers

9. Associations with atrial isomerism

Answers: A B E

Laterality defects are known either as right or left atrial isomerism. Right atrial isomerism (isomerism of the right atrial appendages) is associated with heart defects where both atria are morphologic right atria. Affected children must have anomalous pulmonary venous connection (no left atrium to connect to) by definition. Associated conditions include asplenia, a mid-line liver, malrotation of small bowel, and the presence of two morphologic right lungs. In left atrial isomerism (isomerism of the left atrial appendages), both atria are morphological left atria. Affected children may have anomalous pulmonary venous connections and complex heart disease. It is associated with polysplenia, malrotation and the presence of two morphologic left lungs.

10. Cardiac features of William syndrome

Answers: B E

In William syndrome associated heart defects include supra-valve aortic stenosis and peripheral pulmonary artery stenosis. Other associated defects include a gene abnormality on chromosome 7, hypercalcaemia, serrated teeth, hypertelorism, and cocktail party conversation.

11. Di George syndrome

Answers: B D E

Children with the classical form of Di George syndrome have the chromosomal deletion 22q11.2 plus a heart defect, plus three out of four of the following criteria: absent parathyroids (hypocalcaemia), cleft palate, absent thymus (low T cells) and characteristic facies. Heart defects include interrupted aortic arch, common arterial trunk, tetralogy of Fallot, and familial ventricular septal defect. They should not receive un-irradiated blood transfusion or live vaccines.

12. Kawasaki disease

Answer: A

Kawasaki disease is an acute self-limiting systemic vasculitis of unknown aetiology, which most commonly occurs in children aged 6 months to 5 years. The inflammatory process preferentially involves the coronary arteries, potentially resulting in coronary arteritis, aneurysmal lesions, arterial thrombotic occlusion, and sudden death. Kawasaki disease is the most common cause of acquired coronary vessel abnormalities in children. The diagnosis is based upon recognised clinical criteria, including fever for more than 5 days, and four out of five of the following: mucositis, cervical lymphadenopathy, skin rash, bilateral non-purulent conjunctivitis, and erythema or oedema of the hands and feet. There is no specific diagnostic test to date. Treatment is with intravenous gamma globulin (IVIG 2 g/kg over 12 hours, and high-dose aspirin (30–50 mg/kg/day). It should be initiated as soon as the diagnosis is made, during the febrile period. It is very effective at reducing the incidence of potentially fatal cardiac complications and symptoms attributed to systemic inflammation alike. Coronary artery aneurysms occur in 4.7% of treated cases and 25% of untreated cases.

13. Dilated cardiomyopathy

Answers: All true

Cardiomyopathies are disorders of the heart muscle. In dilated cardiomyopathy, the ventricular size increases whilst the contractility decreases. Mortality is via sudden death or cardiogenic shock and echocardiography shows a globally hypokinetic, dilated heart.

Hypertrophic obstructive cardiomyopathy is a genetic condition with a Mendelian dominant form of inheritance with incomplete penetrance. The most obvious finding on echocardiography is a grossly thickened interventricular septum; the mitral valve also shows a characteristic pattern of apparent systolic anterior motion. Mitochondrial diseases, Friedreich's ataxia, and muscular dystrophies are all associated with cardiomyopathies.

14. Long Q–T interval

Answers: A B D

Causes of a long Q–T interval include:
- Romano–Ward syndrome (autosomal dominant; not lethal)
- Jervell–Lange–Nielsen syndrome (autosomal double dominant; sensorineural deafness; lethal)
- Hypocalcaemia
- Hypokalaemia
- Hypomagnesaemia
- Head injury
- Hypothermia
- Drug administration (such as cisapride or erythromycin)

15. Congenital heart block in fetal life

Answers: A B E

Congenital heart block is usually present from birth. The baby is born with a heart rate of approximately 70 beats/min but is usually not unwell. Often no treatment is required for many years. However, if the affected child fails to thrive, or collapses, develops heart failure, experiences Stokes–Adams attacks, or has a resting heart rate lower than 40/min, intervention should be considered. Causes include maternal systemic lupus erythematosus and congenitally corrected transposition of the great arteries. Of children with congenital complete heart block, 40% have a mother with anti-Ro or anti-La antibodies. Ideally management is expectant. If the child is well and the absolute indications for pacing are not present, then the child should be managed conservatively with 24-hour ECG tapes every few months to document the heart rate. If there are symptoms, or the absolute criteria are satisfied, in-dwelling transvenous pacing should be inserted.

16. Tetralogy of Fallot

Answers: A D E

This condition represents a common form of cyanotic congenital heart disease and encompasses a ventricular septal defect plus sub-pulmonary stenosis plus aorta over-riding the interventricular septum, and as a consequence there is right ventricular hypertrophy. Affected children are usually initially asymptomatic and are rarely severely cyanosed. Presentation is with a loud, harsh ejection systolic murmur at the upper sternal edge on day 1 of life, signifying outflow tract obstruction. The murmur is usually not due to the ventricular septal defect and the children do not usually develop heart failure. Management may be with a systemic-to-pulmonary Blalock–Taussig shunt in the newborn period to increase pulmonary blood flow if severely cyanosed. However, most have elective surgical repair at 6–9 months of age, to close the ventricular septal defect and widen the right ventricular outflow tract.

17. Pulmonary stenosis

Answers: A B D E

In pulmonary stenosis the pulmonary valve leaflets are fused together, giving a restrictive right ventricular outflow tract. The lesion can be valvar, sub-valvar or supra-valvar. Sub-valvar pulmonary stenosis occurs as part of the tetralogy of Fallot. Children are usually asymptomatic and not cyanosed. Investigation involves an assessment with echocardiography, and then balloon dilatation in the catheter laboratory when the gradient reaches 64 mmHg across the valve.

18. Coarctation of the aorta

Answers: D E

Coarctation of the aorta is a duct-dependent narrowing of the aorta, at the point where the ductal tissue encircles the aorta, and thus closes off when the duct closes. It is a common diagnosis, often made antenatally. Children can present with absent femoral pulses, but usually no murmur, and they may be breathless with severe acidosis. They feed poorly, look grey and may be collapsed with a poor peripheral circulation. The liver also enlarges. It is rare for coarctation to present in older children with hypertension and radiofemoral delay. Coarctation is associated with ventricular septal defects in about 10% of cases and a bicuspid aortic valve in 50%.

19. Innocent murmurs

Answers: A B

These are the commonest murmurs heard in children, occurring in up to 50% of normal children. They are often discovered in children with a co-existing infection or with anaemia. Innocent murmurs all relate to a structurally normal heart and it is important to reassure the parents that their child's heart is normal. The types of innocent murmur include those caused by increased flow across the branch pulmonary artery, Still's murmur, and venous hums. The murmur should be soft (no thrill), systolic (diastolic murmurs are not innocent) and short – never pan-systolic. The child is always asymptomatic. The murmur may change with posture (such as venous hums).

20. Noonan syndrome

Answers: A C E

Heart defects include hypertrophic cardiomyopathy, pulmonary valve stenosis, and atrial septal defect. Associated defects include almond-shaped eyes, shallow orbits, a shield-shaped chest with wide spaced nipples and short stature. It is not 'male Turner syndrome' because children with Noonan's may be female and share few of the cardiac similarities.

21. E: Start diuretics and admit to the ward for observation

Ventricular septal defects can be small (restrictive) or large. Small defects occur anywhere in the ventricular septum (peri-membranous or muscular) and do not require imminent cardiac surgery since there is no pulmonary hypertension. About 80–90% of affected children are asymptomatic. They may have a thrill at the left lower sternal edge and have a harsh pan-systolic murmur at the lower left sternal edge with a quiet P2. Large defects occur anywhere in the septum and there is always pulmonary hypertension. Affected children usually become symptomatic with heart failure after 1 week of age; there can be either a soft or no systolic murmur and an apical mid-diastolic heart murmur. They should be treated medically until about 3 months of age, if not in severe heart failure. If the defect is still large at that time, then they should undergo surgical closure. There is usually no need for cardiac catheterisation or magnetic resonance imaging (MRI).

22. D: Pulmonary stenosis

Those children with left-to-right shunts have no signs or symptoms on the first day of life. However, those with outflow obstruction have a murmur from birth. Pulmonary stenosis usually causes no cyanosis, and all neonates have a dominant right ventricle, thus revealing no evidence of right ventricular hypertrophy.

answers

23. B: The baby should be taken to theatre to have a Blalock–Taussig shunt inserted

This condition represents a form of cyanotic congenital heart disease and encompasses a ventricular septal defect plus a sub-pulmonary stenosis with the aorta over-riding the interventricular septum, and hence right ventricular hypertrophy. Affected children are usually asymptomatic and are rarely severely cyanosed. Presentation is with a loud, harsh ejection systolic murmur at the upper sternal edge on day 1 of life, signifying outflow tract obstruction. The murmur is not due to the presence of a ventricular septal defect. These children do not usually develop heart failure. The electrocardiogram is usually normal at birth, but can show right ventricular hypertrophy in older children. The chest radiograph shows an upturned apex in older children (the 'boot-shaped' heart) and a concave left heart border. Oligaemic lung fields are also observed. Management is with a systemic-to-pulmonary Blalock–Taussig shunt in the newborn period to increase pulmonary blood flow if severely cyanosed, but most have elective surgical repair at 6–9 months of age to close the ventricular septal defect and widen the right ventricular outflow tract.

24. D: Ebstein anomaly

Ebstein anomaly is signified by an abnormal and regurgitant tricuspid valve, which is set further down into the right ventricle than normal. The affected child will be cyanosed at birth with a pan-systolic murmur of tricuspid regurgitation at the lower sternal edge. This congenital heart condition has been associated with maternal lithium ingestion.

25. A: Subclavian flap repair for coarctation of the aorta

Coarctation of the aorta is usually a duct-dependent narrowing of the aorta, at the point where the ductal tissue encircles the aorta and thus closes off when the duct closes. It is a common diagnosis, often made antenatally. During the subclavian flap operation to correct the coarctation, the aorta is incised longitudinally across the site of the coarctation and the incision is then extended upwards into the left subclavian artery, which is then ligated and divided. The subclavian flap is brought down as a gusset. This then enlarges the aortic lumen. Following the operation, the left brachial pulse is either very weak or absent but due to a rich collateral blood supply, the left arm continues to grow and will develop normally. There is no interruption to the subclavian artery supply with a pulmonary artery band, a Blalock–Taussig shunt, or an arterial duct ligation.

26. D: Reassure them that the murmur is innocent

This is typical of a venous hum, an innocent heart murmur. It may be easy to hear the venous blood flow returning to the heart, especially at the upper sternal edge. This characteristically occurs in both systole and diastole and disappears when the child lies flat. Innocent murmurs are the commonest murmurs heard in children, occurring in up to 50% of normal children. They are often discovered in children with a co-existing infection or with anaemia. Innocent murmurs all relate to a structurally normal heart and it is clearly important to reassure the parents that their child's heart is normal. Types of innocent murmur include those due to increased flow across the branch pulmonary artery, Still's murmur, and venous hums. The murmur should be soft (no thrill), systolic (diastolic murmurs are not innocent) and short, never pan-systolic. The child is always asymptomatic. The murmur may change with posture, as in venous hums.

27. A: Pompe disease

Pompe disease is a glycogen storage disorder which can affect the heart. It results in an autosomal recessive hypertrophic cardiomyopathy and is rare. Glycogen accumulates in skeletal muscle, the tongue and diaphragm, and in the liver. The heart enlarges as glycogen is deposited in the ventricular muscle. It is a progressive disease. The electrocardiogram reveals a short P–R interval with giant QRS complexes. Chest radiography shows an enlarged heart and often congested lung fields. Treatment is largely supportive.

28. INCIDENCE OF CONGENITAL HEART DISEASE

1.   C – 1 in 1000

There are about 300 children born with hypoplastic left heart syndrome per year.

2.   A – 1 in 100

Congenital heart disease forms the most common group of structural malformations; 8 out of every 1000 live births have congenital heart disease.

3.   B – 1 in 500

Ventricular septal defect occurs in 30% of children with congenital heart disease. Congenital heart disease forms the most common group of structural malformations; eight out of every 1000 live births have congenital heart disease. There are eight or nine common lesions that account for about 80% of all cases. The remaining 20% encompass a multitude of complex lesions. There are about 300 children born with hypoplastic left heart syndrome each year. The more common lesions can be subdivided as follows, in order of incidence:

- Ventricular septal defect 30%
- Persistent arterial duct 12%
- Atrial septal defect 7%
- Pulmonary stenosis 7%
- Aortic stenosis 5%
- Coarctation of the aorta 5%
- Tetralogy of Fallot 5%
- Transposition of the great arteries 5%
- Atrioventricular septal defect 2%

answers

Incidence is increased by a positive family history of coronary heart disease:
- Previous sibling with coronary heart disease 2%
- Two siblings with coronary heart disease 4%
- Father with coronary heart disease 3%
- Mother with coronary heart disease 6%.

29. PRESENTATIONS OF CONGENITAL HEART DISEASE

1. G: Transposition of the great arteries
The presentation of a baby with cardiac disease at 2 days of age suggests a duct-dependent lesion. Severe cyanosis is most often caused by transposition of the great arteries, where there is usually no murmur, but the second sound is single (aorta in front of the pulmonary artery) and there is heart failure due to acidosis.

2. D: Hypoplastic left heart syndrome
The differential diagnosis in a baby with collapse at 2 days of age and not cyanotic is obstructed left heart (coarctation, hypoplastic left heart syndrome, critical aortic stenosis or interrupted aortic arch), metabolic acidosis, or sepsis. All of these should be considered, but the absence of all pulses make hypoplastic left heart or critical aortic stenosis the most likely. Hypoplastic left heart syndrome is much more common of the two.

3. A: Atrial septal defect
Ejection systolic murmurs at the upper left sternal edge in asymptomatic children are most likely to be innocent, or an atrial septal defect, or pulmonary stenosis, or arterial ducts. In this child with a split S2 and the ECG findings, atrial septal defect is the most likely.

30. DYSRHYTHMIAS

1. C: Intravenous adenosine
In the management of supraventricular tachycardia the goal is to terminate the episode and restore sinus rhythm. A narrow complex tachycardia with a rate of > 240 beats/minute is likely to be seen on the electrocardiogram. Vagal manoeuvres could be attempted first, such as applying an ice pack to the face, carotid sinus massage, or by intravenous adenosine 50–250 µg/kg, and finally DC synchronised cardioversion 0.5–2.0 J/kg. Prophylaxis for arrhythmias tends to differ between cardiac units. However, for supraventricular tachycardia they include digoxin and propranolol, flecainide or sotalol.

2. F: Defibrillation
To manage ventricular tachycardia, synchronised cardioversion at 0.5–2.0 J/kg should be attempted if a pulse is present. If no pulse is present, then defibrillation should be used at 2–4 J/kg. If a child is alternating between sinus rhythm and ventricular tachycardia, then an infusion of amiodarone is safest and most effective. Prophylaxis for arrhythmias tends to differ between cardiac units. However, for ventricular tachycardia they include flecainide, sotalol and amiodarone (beware of toxicity to the thyroid, skin and lungs).

3.　G: Radiofrequency ablation

Once a child reaches about 4 years old, then ongoing prophylaxis may be disruptive on his or her lifestyle. Radiofreqency ablation can then be offered.

Child development, child psychiatry and community paediatrics

Jo Philpot

Multiple Choice Questions

1. In a normal 12-month-old infant

- ○ A the Moro reflex is absent
- ○ B the parachute reflex is absent
- ○ C the stepping reflex is present
- ○ D the asymmetrical tonic neck reflex is present
- ○ E the head-righting reflex is absent

2. A typical 4-year-old is able to

- ○ A skip
- ○ B copy a square
- ○ C dress with supervision
- ○ D draw a person with six parts
- ○ E write their name

3. The following are risk factors for sudden infant death syndrome

- ○ A male sex
- ○ B age 16–30 weeks
- ○ C maternal age above 35 years
- ○ D maternal smoking
- ○ E supine sleeping position

4. It is safe for HIV-infected children to have the following immunisations

- ○ A measles–mumps–rubella (MMR)
- ○ B bacille Calmette–Guérin (BCG)
- ○ C *Haemophilus influenzae* type B (HIB)
- ○ D diphtheria–pertussis–tetanus (DPT)
- ○ E hepatitis B

5. A typical 2-year-old is able to

- ○ A copy a circle
- ○ B point to three body parts
- ○ C say 50 words
- ○ D name three colours
- ○ E jump well

6. The following statements about attention deficit hyperactivity disorder are correct

- ○ A it is commoner in boys
- ○ B a history of marked hyperactivity for 6 months' duration should be present before making the diagnosis
- ○ C the diagnosis should be made before school entry if possible
- ○ D once treatment with methylphenidate hydrochloride (Ritalin) is commenced, educational support is rarely needed
- ○ E hypotension is a recognised side effect of Ritalin

7. Risk factors for suicide in adolescents are

- ○ A female sex
- ○ B alcohol addiction
- ○ C immigrant status
- ○ D family history of suicide
- ○ E no previous suicide attempt

8. The following disorders are associated with developmental delay

- ○ A Tay–Sachs disease
- ○ B Marfan syndrome
- ○ C Prader–Willi syndrome
- ○ D spinal muscular atrophy
- ○ E Duchenne muscular dystrophy

9. A healthy 12-month-old should be able to

- ○ A wave bye-bye
- ○ B feed with a spoon
- ○ C point to a body part
- ○ D transfer an object from one hand to another
- ○ E walk

10. The measles–mumps–rubella (MMR) vaccine is

- ○ A contraindicated in children with egg allergy
- ○ B a live vaccine
- ○ C contraindicated in children with autistic spectrum disorder
- ○ D recognised as having more side effects after the second dose
- ○ E contraindicated in a child with Di George syndrome

11. Medical complications of anorexia include

- ○ A hypercholesterolaemia
- ○ B lanugo
- ○ C amenorrhoea
- ○ D thrombocytopenia
- ○ E constipation

12. In the cover test

- ○ A the fixation object needs to be 1 metre away
- ○ B if the uncovered eye does not move when the other eye is covered, no squint is present
- ○ C if the uncovered eye moves towards the nose (temporally) to fix on the object when the other eye is covered, a manifest convergent squint is present
- ○ D a pseudosquint cannot be diagnosed from a true squint
- ○ E the child should be older than 2 years for the results to be accurate

13. Tympanometry

- ○ A is not useful in children aged under 18 months
- ○ B is not helpful in the diagnosis of 'glue ear'
- ○ C shows a peak at 0 pressure if there is Eustachian tube dysfunction
- ○ D shows a flattened trace if a middle-ear effusion is present
- ○ E needs to be repeated after 3 months to confirm the diagnosis

14. In autistic spectrum disorder

- ○ A boys outnumber girls by 3 to 1
- ○ B associated intellectual impairment is common
- ○ C the diagnosis is usually made before the age of 3 years
- ○ D the brain MRI scan often shows non-specific white matter changes
- ○ E an electroencephalogram (EEG) should be performed to exclude epilepsy

15. A typical 3-year-old is able to

- ○ A count to 10
- ○ B copy a cross
- ○ C stand on one foot
- ○ D draw a person with three parts
- ○ E name three colours

Best of Five Questions

16. A 3-year-old boy is referred to the outpatient department with concerns about his development. The pregnancy and neonatal history were uneventful and he has had no serious illnesses. He has always been slow with his development. His mother also had mild learning difficulties and needed extra help in school. On assessment he can walk but cannot jump. He has poor eye contact, has no clear words and cannot identify parts of his body. He is unable to copy a horizontal line and is still in nappies. Examination is very difficult because he becomes very distressed and demonstrates hand flapping. His head circumference is on the 90th centile. Which of the following is the MOST useful investigation?

○ A Thyroid studies
○ B MRI brain scan
○ C Urinary organic acids
○ D Genetic studies
○ E Electroencephalogram (EEG)

17. A 3-year-old boy is referred to the outpatient department with concerns about speech and language development. The pregnancy and neonatal history were uneventful and he has had no serious illnesses. At 15 months he had five clear words that he has since stopped using. He enjoys puzzles, is able to feed using a spoon and fork, and can dress himself with help. There has been difficulty settling him into nursery. He becomes very distressed and runs around being disruptive and sometimes physically aggressive towards other children. On assessment he is very difficult to settle and tries to escape from the room. He does not demonstrate any clear words or understanding of simple commands and refuses to engage in any activities. Which of the following is the MOST likely diagnosis?

○ A Attention deficit disorder
○ B Specific speech and language delay
○ C Autistic spectrum disorder
○ D Deafness
○ E Global developmental delay

18. A 14-year-old girl is seen in clinic with a history of a severe sore throat and fever 4 months ago. Since then she has had headaches, generalised muscle pain, tiredness, and poor concentration of increasing severity. For the past 2 months she has been unable to attend school because of her muscle pain and lethargy, and her sleep pattern has become disturbed. She finds it very difficult to fall asleep at night and then has difficulty getting up in the morning. On examination she has mild lymphadenopathy and looks pale. Her weight is continuing along the 25th centile. Examination is otherwise unremarkable except for the marked muscle pain she experiences on movement of her limbs. Which of the following is the MOST likely diagnosis?

    ○ A Depression
    ○ B Chronic fatigue syndrome
    ○ C Hypothyroidism
    ○ D Crohn's disease
    ○ E Anorexia nervosa

19. A 13-year-old girl is seen in clinic with a history of weight loss over the past 6 months. Her weight has gone from the 75th to the 3rd centile and her height has continued along the 50th. Apart from her periods, which have stopped, her general health has been fine. She is in the county's gymnastic squad, but over the last 2 months she has missed training sessions. Her examination is unremarkable. Which of the following is the MOST likely diagnosis?

    ○ A Depression
    ○ B Chronic fatigue syndrome
    ○ C Hyperthyroidism
    ○ D Crohn's disease
    ○ E Anorexia nervosa

20. A 15-month-old child is seen in clinic with a 3-month history of collapsing. The episodes occur when he has been hurt. He suddenly looks very pale, loses consciousness, and falls to the floor. He then appears to stiffen and has some clonic movements of his arms and legs before quickly recovering. Examination is unremarkable. Which of the following is the MOST likely diagnosis?

    ○ A Prolonged QT syndrome
    ○ B Reflex anoxic seizures
    ○ C Complex partial epilepsy
    ○ D Tonic–clonic seizures
    ○ E Myoclonic seizures

questions

Extended Matching Questions

21. Theme: Developmental delay

A   Wood's light
B   Genetic studies for Angelman syndrome
C   Genetic studies for spinal muscular atrophy
D   Genetic studies for fragile X
E   Creatine kinase
F   Serum lactate
G   Urine for glycosaminoglycans
H   Genetic studies for Prader–Willi

For each patient below, select the most appropriate investigation from the list above: Each option may be used once, more than once, or not at all.

○ 1. A 3-year-old with seizures and severe developmental delay who has ataxia and jerky movements on clinical examination.

○ 2. A 4-month-old presenting with infantile spasms.

○ 3. A neonate with a birth weight below the 3rd centile with hypotonia and a weak suck requiring nasogastric feeding.

22. Theme: Speech delay

A   Electroencephalogram (EEG)
B   Urine organic acids
C   Creatine kinase
D   Brain MRI
E   Hearing assessment
F   Lactate
G   Genetic studies for fragile X
H   Electrocardiogram (ECG)
I   Ammonia

For each patient below, select the most appropriate investigation from those listed above. Each option may be used once, more than once, or not at all.

○ 1. A 3-year-old boy presents with loss of language skills. Speech development appeared to be normal until his third birthday, following which he has become progressively more aphasic.

○ 2. A 3-year-old boy presents with delay in expressive speech and comprehension. Questioning reveals that he walked at 18 months and had his first clear word at 2 years. His eye contact is normal but it is difficult to keep him on task. On developmental assessment he can copy vertical lines but not a circle. He can identify animals in a book and one colour. Expressively he is not putting two words together. He is still wearing nappies.

○ 3. A 3-year-old boy presents with delay in expressive speech and comprehension. On questioning, he walked at 24 months and had his first clear word at 2 years. His eye contact is poor and it is very difficult to keep him on task. On developmental assessment he can scribble but prefers fiddling with the crayons and chewing them. He cannot point to parts of his body and grunts in response to questions. No clear words are demonstrated. He is still wearing nappies. He has an uncle, now aged 28, who is known to have developmental delay and was very slow to walk.

23. Theme: Children Act

A   Place of Safety Order
B   Care Order
C   Wardship
D   Child Assessment Order
E   Supervision Order
F   Police Protection Order
G   Emergency Protection Order (EPO)
H   Statementing Order

Identify the following orders of the Children Act 1989 below from those listed above. Each option may be used once, more than once, or not at all.

○ 1. This order lasts for a maximum of 8 days with a possibility of extension for a further 7 days. This order may be granted by the court if there is reason to believe a child may be harmed if not removed from their present accommodation.

○ 2. This order confers parental responsibility on the social services (in addition to that of the parents) and usually involves removal from home. It may be applied for in cases of non-accidental injury where inquires will take some time and where the child is not regarded as being safe at home.

○ 3. This order may be used if there is a situation of persistent but non-urgent suspicion of risk. It overrides the objections of a parent to whatever examination or assessment is needed to see whether the child is at significant harm. This order lasts up to 7 days.

answers

1. Normal 12-month-old infants

Answer: A

The primitive reflexes are stereotyped responses that disappear in a predictable order as the child matures. The Moro reflex is present from birth to 4 months. Asymmetry of the Moro reflex occurs in brachial plexus injury and fracture of the clavicle. Persistence of the Moro can be an early sign of cerebral palsy. The parachute reflex develops at around 9 months of age. It consists of extension of the hands and arms when the infant in the prone position is allowed to fall a short distance. This protective reflex persists for life. The stepping reflex is present at birth and disappears at 6 weeks. The asymmetrical tonic neck reflex disappears around 6 months of age. Its persistence occurs in children with cerebral palsy. The head-righting reflex develops at 6 months of age and persists.

2. Typical 4-year-olds

Answers: B C

Typical 4-year-old children can jump and are starting to hop, but are usually unable to skip. They can copy a square and a cross but not a triangle. They can draw a person with three parts and dress with supervision. A 5-year-old can typically write their name and draw a person with six parts.

3. Sudden infant death syndrome

Answers: A D

Many hypotheses have developed about the causes of sudden infant death syndrome (SIDS). The search for an individual cause has shifted to a more complex model. It seems likely that SIDS is due to an interaction of risk factors – developmental stage, congenital and acquired risks, and a final trigger. Established risk factors for SIDS are: age 4–16 weeks, prone and side-sleeping position, overheating, soft sleeping surfaces, fever/minor infection, bed-sharing with parents, maternal smoking (ante- and postnatal), low maternal age, low birth weight, pre-term delivery, medical complications in the neonatal period, social deprivation, male sex, and inborn errors of metabolism.

4. Immunisation of HIV-infected children

Answers: A C D E

Current recommendations are that it is safe for HIV-infected children to receive: MMR, oral polio (inactivated form may be given), pertussis, diphtheria, tetanus, typhoid, cholera, hepatitis B and HIB. They should not have BCG, yellow fever and oral typhoid.

5. Typical 2-year-olds

Answers: B C

Children of 2 years old are able to express at least 50 words and point to several body parts. They are also able to climb over furniture and are starting to go up and down stairs one step at a time. Copying a circle, naming three colours, and jumping are skills found in a typical 3-year-old.

6. Attention deficit hyperactivity disorder

Answer: A

It is estimated that 1% of school-age children in the UK meet the diagnostic criteria for attention deficit hyperactivity disorder (ADHD). It is characterized by problems with inattention, hyperactivity and impulsiveness. The behaviour should have been present for at least 6 months but not all three features have to be present (for example, it is possible to have marked inattention without the hyperactivity). Management involves a comprehensive treatment programme and close communication with the school is vital. Ritalin does not cure ADHD but improves the symptoms to allow other behavioural interventions an opportunity to take effect.

7. Suicide in adolescents

Answers: B C D

Suicide is rare before puberty, yet it is the third leading cause of death for adolescents with rates in young men continuing to rise. Methods include drug overdose, hanging, inhalation of car exhaust fumes and shooting. It is by far the minority of adolescents who make suicide attempts who have either an underlying psychiatric disorder or serious suicidal intent. All individuals who make a suicide attempt must undergo psychiatric assessment. The use of violent methods, attempts which take place in isolated places, and the writing of a suicide note should ring particular alarm bells. Risk factors for suicide in adolescents include: male sex, broken home, disturbed relationships with parents, living alone, immigrant status, family history of affective disorder, suicide or alcohol abuse, recent loss or stress, previous suicide attempt, drug or alcohol addiction. Although suicide is commoner in males, deliberate self harm such as poisoning and self-mutilation is much commoner in females.

8. Developmental delay

Answers: A C E

Muscle disorders associated with developmental delay include Duchenne muscular dystrophy and myotonic dystrophy. Tay–Sachs disease is a neurodegenerative disease of the grey matter with most children dying between 3 to 4 years of age. Developmental delay is not a feature of Marfan syndrome or spinal muscular atrophy.

answers

9. Healthy 12-month-olds

Answers: A D

Waving bye-bye develops around 10 months of age, and transferring at 6 months. Pointing to body parts and spoon-feeding occur at around 18 months. Although children do walk at 12 months most are still cruising. They should be walking by 18 months.

10. MMR vaccine

Answers: B E

The MMR vaccine is a live vaccine and therefore is contraindicated in children with impaired cell-mediated immunity, as in Di George syndrome. Other contraindications for live vaccines include prednisolone (orally or rectally) at a daily dose of 2 mg/kg per day for at least 1 week or 1 mg/kg per day for a month, lower doses of steroid if used in conjunction with cytotoxic drugs, immunosuppression secondary to an underlying disease, immunoglobulin administration in the previous 6 months, children who have had a bone marrow transplant within 6 months and children being treated for malignant disease with chemotherapy/radiotherapy or who have completed treatment in the past 6 months. MMR is not contraindicated in egg allergy or in children with autistic spectrum disorder. Side effects include malaise, fever, rash within 7–10 days, parotid swelling 1%, febrile convulsion 1/1000. Arthropathy/thrombocytopenia are rare. All side effects are less common after the second dose.

11. Complications of anorexia

Answer: All true

Anorexia has become increasingly recognised in paediatric practice. Over 90% of those affected are female. Medical complications include:

Central nervous system
- Reversible cortical atrophy
- Non-specific EEG abnormalities

Dental
- Caries
- Periodontitis

Pulmonary
- Aspiration pneumonia (rare)

Cardiovascular
- Bradycardia
- Hypotension
- Arrhythmias
- Cardiomyopathy (rare)

Gastrointestinal
- Parotitis
- Delayed gastric emptying
- Gastric dilatation
- Constipation
- Raised amylase (bulimia)

Renal/electrolyte
- Hypokalaemia
- Hypochloraemic metabolic alkalosis
- Oedema
- Renal calculi (rare)

Neuroendocrine
- Amenorrhoea
- Oligomenorrhea (bulimia)

Musculoskeletal
- Myopathy
- Osteoporosis and pathological fractures

Haematological
- Anaemia
- Thrombocytopenia
- Hypercholesterolaemia
- Hypercarotenaemia

Dermatological
- Dry, cracking skin
- Lanugo
- Callous on dorsum of hand (from vomiting)
- Peri-oral dermatitis

Some 5–10 years after the diagnosis of anorexia nervosa around 50% will have recovered, 25% will have improved but still have some features of an eating disorder, and the remainder will either not have improved or be dead. Mortality rates are around 5% but may rise further with longer term follow up.

12. Cover test

Answer: C

In the cover test both eyes need to be tested before deciding that no squint is present. It can distinguish a true squint from a pseudosquint. The squinting eye takes up fixation of the object when the other eye is covered. When the cover is removed the squinting eye returns to its original position. A manifest squint is present all the time. A latent squint is only present at times of stress (eg tiredness). If the eye turns inwards, it is convergent; if it turns outwards, it is divergent.

13. Tympanometry

Answer: D

Tympanometry assesses the compliance of the tympanic membrane and ear ossicles. It is suitable for children of any age and is primarily used to check for glue ear. In the normal ear the peak is at 0 pressure, reflecting equal pressures on either side of the drum. In a middle-ear effusion the trace is flattened.

14. Autistic spectrum disorder

Answers: A B

Studies suggest that autism is becoming more common. Although abnormal function is observed before 3 years of age, the diagnosis is not usually made until the child is over 3. There is no consensus regarding appropriate investigations such as chromosomes, brain MRI and EEG, which are usually all normal. Some perform MRI, EEGs and chromosomal studies routinely. Others only perform the tests if there is a clinical indication: for example, chromosomes if dysmorphic features are found; EEG if there are variations in symptoms or developmental regression to rule out subclinical epilepsy and epilepsy syndromes such as Landau–Kleffner.

15. Typical 3-year-olds

Answer: E

A 3-year-old can identify three colours, copy a circle, and jump. Copying a cross, standing on one foot, drawing a person with three parts and counting to 10 is typical of a 4-year-old.

16. D: Genetic studies

The history tells us that the child is a boy with a mother with learning difficulties. This should always raise the concern regarding fragile X and Duchenne muscular dystrophy. The examination reveals a child with significant developmental delay, autistic features and a large head, all in keeping with a diagnosis of fragile X. The other investigations are reasonable in a child with developmental delay but in this case are less likely to provide a diagnosis.

17. C: Autistic spectrum disorder

From the history some of his development is age appropriate, excluding global developmental delay. The history and his behaviour in clinic makes specific speech and language delay and deafness unlikely. Attention deficit disorder is a possibility but it would not explain his regression of language at around 15 months of age and the severe delay in speech and language since. It is also unusual to make a diagnosis of attention deficit disorder in such a young child. Autistic spectrum disorder would explain all the findings and is the most likely diagnosis.

18. B: Chronic fatigue syndrome

The lack of weight loss excludes anorexia nervosa and makes Crohn's disease unlikely. If hypothyroidism was severe enough to cause her to take 2 months off school, her weight would have been expected to rise, thus excluding hypothyroidism as a diagnosis. Depression is a possibility but the sleep pattern is not typical. Chronic fatigue syndrome often develops after a viral illness. Headaches, generalised muscle pains, poor concentration and sleep disturbance are all features of the illness. Pallor and mild cervical ' lymphadenopathy are common. Weight is usually static or can increase slightly due to lack of exercise by the individual.

19. E: Anorexia nervosa

Anorexia is the most likely diagnosis. Crohn's disease is a possibility but there is no history of any bowel disturbance despite a dramatic loss in weight. If she had hyperthyroidism there should have been some clinical signs on examination, such as tachycardia, sweaty palms, or goitre. The history is also not typical of chronic fatigue syndrome.

20. B: Reflex anoxic seizures

Although the child appears to stiffen and has some clonic movements of his limbs, complex partial epilepsy, tonic–clonic seizures, and myoclonic seizures are unlikely as the events are always after a stimulus, and because he looks pale and there is a quick recovery.

21. DEVELOPMENTAL DELAY

1.   B – Genetic studies for Angelman syndrome

Angelman syndrome (previously known as happy puppet syndrome) is caused by a deletion of chromosome 15q11.2–12 which is maternally inherited. Clinical features include severe learning difficulty, ataxia, jerky movements, seizures and a cheerful demeanour.

2.   A – Wood's light

There are many causes of infantile spasms. In 10–15% no cause is found (cryptogenic) and these cases are more likely to run a more favourable course. Brain dysgenesis and neurocutaneous syndromes (mainly tuberous sclerosis) are the most frequently identified causes of infantile spasms. Tuberous sclerosis accounts for 10–20% of cases and therefore examining with a Wood's light to identify hypomelanotic macules would be the investigation of choice from the ones listed above, and it is easy to perform.

3.   H – Genetic studies for Prader–Willi

According to the description the neonate has a neuromuscular disorder, which means that answers C, E and H are possible. The presentation is too early for Duchenne muscular dystrophy, eliminating answer C. Neonates with spinal muscular atrophy are hypotonic but characteristically the facial muscles are spared and feeding problems are very unusual. Babies with

answers

Prader–Willi are often of low birth weight despite the tendency in older life to become obese. They present in the neonatal period with hypotonia and feeding difficulties, and therefore answer H is correct.

22. SPEECH DELAY

1. A – Electroencephalogram (EEG)

The diagnosis of Landau–Kleffner syndrome should be considered in a child who loses language skills. The onset is usually between 3 years and 9 years and is characterized by rapid loss of language skills after initial normal language development. There are typical EEG abnormalities, and it has a variable prognosis. Most patients will still have language difficulties as adults ranging from those with almost no verbal ability to those with mild deficits in verbal communication.

2. C – Creatine kinase

This child is showing mild delay in all areas of his development, more marked in speech and language. The diagnosis that needs to be excluded is Duchenne muscular dystrophy, particularly as he only walked at 18 months. Boys with Duchenne muscular dystrophy usually have associated learning difficulties and often present to the medical professional with concerns about speech and language before any muscle weakness is apparent.

3. G – Genetic studies for fragile X

This child is showing significant developmental delay in all areas of his development. He is also demonstrating some autistic features with poor eye contact, chewing, and fiddling. The information about the uncle suggests a genetic disease such as fragile X. Duchenne muscular dystrophy is not likely as affected individuals do not usually survive into their late 20s.

23. CHILDREN ACT

1. G – Emergency Protection Order (EPO)

This replaced the Place of Safety Order and may be granted by the court if one of the following is satisfied:

- There is reasonable cause to believe that the child is likely to suffer appreciable harm if not removed from their present accommodation.
- Inquiries by the local authority are being frustrated by lack of access. In addition a child likely to suffer significant harm may also be taken into police protection for 72 hours; this involves a decision internal to the police force and is quicker than applying for an EPO.

2. B – Care Order

Care orders may be taken out by a court if they are convinced that the threshold for appreciable harm to the child has been met.

3. D – Child Assessment Order

A Child Assessment Order may be used if there is a situation of persistent but non-urgent suspicion of risk. A Supervision Order gives the social services the power and duty to visit the family and also to impose conditions, such as attendance at a clinic, nursery, school, or outpatients visits.

If insufficient powers are available via the Children Act then Wardship via the High Court may be applied for. This gives the court virtually unlimited powers and is used in exceptional circumstances, such as when a family objects to medical treatment because of religious reasons. The Statementing Order does not exist.

answers

Clinical pharmacology and toxicology

Stephen Tomlin and Michael Capra

Multiple Choice Questions

1. Bioavailability of an oral acidic drug is dependent on

○ A the formulation of the drug
○ B the rate of excretion
○ C the acidity of the stomach
○ D plasma concentration of the drug
○ E the dose that has been taken

2. Neonatal gastric absorption often differs from that of adults due to the following factors

○ A they have no functional villi
○ B the gastric pH is higher than adults
○ C gastric motility is decreased
○ D neonates only absorb from the stomach and not the intestines
○ E meconium creates a barrier to absorption

3. Concerning drug volumes of distribution

○ A at birth the percentage of total body water is increased
○ B the extracellular fluid volume is increased in newborn babies
○ C water soluble drugs have a lower volume of distribution in newborn babies than adolescents
○ D benzylpenicillin is required in higher doses on a mg/kg basis in a child compared to a neonate to achieve the same plasma concentration
○ E newborn babies have a smaller volume of distribution for fat soluble drugs than infants

4. Concerning protein binding of phenytoin in neonates

○ A phenytoin does not bind to protein in neonates
○ B protein binding is decreased due to the decreased phenytoin plasma levels
○ C total plasma levels are lower due to increased albumin binding
○ D therapeutic drug levels are lower than for adults due to increased amounts of non-protein-bound phenytoin
○ E neonates have a decreased binding capacity for phenytoin compared to adults

5. Concerning drug penetration of the blood–brain barrier (BBB)

○ A diazepam is fat soluble and readily crosses the BBB
○ B the more ionised a drug is the faster it will get into the cerebrospinal fluid
○ C neonates have increased absorption of opiates across the BBB
○ D sulfonamides increase the bilirubin displacement from albumin and thus can help treat kernicterus
○ E gentamicin easily penetrates the BBB and thus is suitable for Gram-negative encephalitis

6. Concerning the half-life of drugs

○ A equal quantities of drug are excreted in each successive half-life
○ B drugs are said to be in steady state after 4–5 doses
○ C loading doses decrease the time to steady state
○ D drugs with very short half-lives should be given by intermittent injection to ensure a steady plasma level
○ E half-lives indicate peak plasma level times

7. Concerning neonatal hepatic metabolism

○ A the half-life of diazepam is increased in neonates due to decreased hepatic metabolism
○ B grey baby syndrome is a rare toxic effect of chloramphenicol due to decreased neonatal hepatic glucuronidation
○ C Paracetamol is mainly sulfated in neonates because the usual glucuronidation process is not developed
○ D caffeine is used as a respiratory stimulant in neonates as it has a higher therapeutic efficacy than theophylline
○ E gentamicin is metabolised in the liver in neonates, but is cleared renally in children.

8. In severe renal failure

○ A the dose of digoxin needs to be reduced
○ B cephalosporins are much safer than penicillin in high dose
○ C sucralfate is the antacid of choice

○ D aminoglycosides are always given once daily
○ E peritoneal dialysis is less effective than haemodialysis at reducing blood levels

9 Concerning systemic lupus erythematosus (SLE)

○ A slow acetylators have an increased risk of SLE
○ B drug-induced SLE occurs in all children who cannot metabolise isoniazid
○ C isoniazid may induce SLE
○ D phenytoin may induce SLE
○ E penicillin may induce SLE

10. The following is true for children with impaired liver function

○ A the respiratory depressant effect of morphine is decreased
○ B plasma potassium levels are more likely to decrease when using loop diuretics
○ C patients are more likely to bleed if being treated with warfarin
○ D cyclosporin causes renal impairment, so doses do not need to be decreased, nor monitoring increased, in liver impairment
○ E patients may become phenytoin-toxic even if their plasma levels remain in the therapeutic range

11. In therapeutic drug monitoring

○ A plasma vancomycin levels can be used to monitor efficacy and toxicity
○ B plasma gentamicin levels should not be < 1 mg/L before the next dose
○ C hypokalaemia can predispose a child to digoxin toxicity even if the plasma drug level is within the recommended range
○ D phenytoin levels are best taken after the third dose
○ E carbamazepine plasma levels should remain constant after 1 week of treatment

12. Regarding accidental ingestion of iron by a child

○ A symptoms of abdominal pain, nausea and vomiting may occur approximately 8 hours following ingestion
○ B toxicity is likely if the total ingested dose of elemental iron exceeds 250 mg/kg
○ C in an untreated case of toxic iron ingestion, hepatic failure and hypoglycaemia occur 2–4 days after ingestion
○ D desferrioxamine administered orally or intravenously may be effective in limiting toxicity
○ E an abdominal X-ray is of limited use because elemental iron is not radio-opaque

questions

13. Regarding toxic ingestion/ inhalation of substances

○ A acute salicylate ingestion causes a metabolic alkalosis

○ B induced emesis is contraindicated when a corrosive substance is ingested

○ C acute lead poisoning may lead to behavioural and cognitive disturbances

○ D tricyclic antidepressants may cause urinary retention, dry mouth and constricted pupils

○ E carbon monoxide poisoning causes tissue hypoxia despite a normal PaO_2

Best of Five Questions

14. A pre-term neonate who weighs 2.5 kg and is 3 days old requires a higher dose of benzylpenicillin on a mg/kg basis than an adult to achieve the same plasma concentration. Which of the following BEST describes why this should be?

- ○ A Benzylpenicillin crosses the blood–brain barrier in neonates more readily
- ○ B Neonates have a higher volume of distribution for water-soluble drugs
- ○ C Benzylpenicillin is water soluble and distributes to the kidneys at a faster rate in neonates
- ○ D Benzylpenicillin is excreted from the kidney more slowly in neonates
- ○ E The protein binding of benzylpenicillin is lower in neonates

15. The therapeutic plasma range of phenytoin is lower in neonates than in children. What is the MOST likely reason for this?

- ○ A Less phenytoin is needed to treat seizures on a mg/kg basis
- ○ B Bilirubin displaces phenytoin from albumin more readily in neonates
- ○ C Decreased albumin levels lead to increased free phenytoin
- ○ D Phenytoin is more toxic in neonates
- ○ E Phenytoin is excreted more slowly in neonates

16. Chloramphenicol may cause 'grey baby syndrome' in neonates. What is the MOST likely reason for this?

- ○ A Chloramphenicol is able to cross the blood–brain barrier
- ○ B Neonatal livers are unable to glucuronidate high doses of chloramphenicol
- ○ C Chloramphenicol is glucuronidated to a toxic metabolite in neonates
- ○ D Grey baby syndrome is an idiosyncratic reaction of chloramphenicol in neonates
- ○ E Neonatal sulphation is more established at birth than glucuronidation

17. A neonate born at 37/40 who is 2 weeks old was commenced on phenytoin 2 days ago. A plasma level of phenytoin taken 8 hours post-dose was 8 mg/L and the patient is still having seizures. What would be the MOST appropriate clinical approach?

- ○ A Leave the prescription the same because steady state hasn't been reached
- ○ B Double the dose and monitor in another 3 days
- ○ C Increase the dose by about 20% and monitor the child
- ○ D Monitor the albumin to see if it is a true level
- ○ E Stop the phenytoin and start another anticonvulsant

questions

18. A 10-kg 14-month-old boy is brought to the accident and emergency department by his parents. His parents claim that he possibly ingested paracetamol, as six 500 mg capsules were found to be missing from the family's paracetamol container. This possible ingestion occurred within a 60 minute window prior to their presentation to the A & E department. Which is the MOST appropriate immediate management action of the five choices below?

- ○ A Measure plasma paracetamol levels
- ○ B Administer ipecacuanha to induce emesis
- ○ C Perform a gastric lavage
- ○ D Administer *N*-acetylcysteine
- ○ E Administer activated charcoal

Extended Matching Questions

19. Theme: Neonatal pharmacokinetics

- ○ A Gut motility
- ○ B Gut acidity
- ○ C Hepatic glucuronidation
- ○ D Hepatic sulphation
- ○ E Renal function
- ○ F Protein binding
- ○ G Volume of distribution
- ○ II Permeability of blood-brain barrier

Select the process which is most likely to be altered (from that of children and adults) to be responsible for the following situations in neonates. Each option may be used once, more than once, or not at all.

- ○ 1. A 2-week-old term baby requires a higher dose (on a mg/kg basis) of a water-soluble drug in order to achieve the same plasma concentration.
- ○ 2. The neonate generally has a lower therapeutic range than adults and children for phenytoin.
- ○ 3. Dosing of benzylpenicillin in a 1-week-old, 30-week gestation neonate is usually at a frequency of two or three times a day-as opposed to four times a day in children.

20. Theme: Therapeutic drug monitoring

- ○ A Phenytoin
- ○ B Carbamazepine
- ○ C Phenobarbitone
- ○ D Digoxin
- ○ E Warfarin
- ○ F Gentamicin
- ○ G Vancomycin
- ○ H Theophylline

For each of the scenarios below, which of the listed drugs is most likely to be implicated. Each option may be used once, more than once, or not at all.

- ○ 1. The plasma levels of this drug have been rising over the last 2 weeks but are now falling (the dose has remained the same).
- ○ 2. An infant has had her drug dose increased by 25% every 5 days and the plasma levels have been increasing slowly, but levels are still just below the therapeutic range. Five days after the next 25% increase the infant's levels are above the therapeutic range, with symptoms of toxicity.

○ 3. A child who has had appropriate plasma levels for several years is now able to take tablets instead of liquid. On changing the preparation (but keeping the dose the same) the plasma levels taken 2 weeks after the change are sub-therapeutic.

answers

1. Bioavailability of oral acidic drugs

Answers: A C

Bioavailability is applied to the rate and extent of the drug absorption. It is thus dependent on the chemical make-up of the drug, and the form into which it is transformed within the acidic gut. Drugs are absorbed in their non-ionised state and thus acidic medication will generally be absorbed more readily within the gut.

2. Neonatal gastric absorption

Answers: B C

Soon after birth, acid is released into the stomach; however the pH of the stomach remains higher than in adulthood until 2–3 years of life. Since most drugs are either basic or acidic the amount of ionisation will vary in neonates and thus absorption will vary. Gastric motility is also decreased during infancy, thus increasing the absorption of drugs which are absorbed in the stomach. Villi are present at birth and meconium should not cause a problem.

3. Drug volumes of distribution

Answers: A B E

Newborn babies have very little fat and a high proportion of extracellular fluid. Water-soluble drugs such as benzylpenicillin therefore have a higher volume of distribution in neonates and require higher doses on a mg/kg basis to achieve the same plasma concentrations. Fat-soluble drugs have a lower volume of distribution in newborns than in adults, but this usually reverses by the time they reach 1 year of age.

4. Protein binding of phenytoin

Answers: D E

Phenytoin is a highly protein-bound drug. Neonates have lower levels of protein than adults, and the protein they do have binds albumin less tightly. Thus neonates have more non-bound phenytoin, which is the active component. Plasma levels of phenytoin measure total phenytoin and thus therapeutic ranges are lower in neonates as a greater percentage is active.

5. Drugs and the blood–brain barrier

Answers: A C

Fat-soluble and non-ionised drugs (those with no positive or negative charge) penetrate the blood–brain barrier (BBB) more rapidly and more easily than water-soluble and ionised drugs. Neonates have a functionally incomplete BBB and hence there is an increased penetration of some drugs into the brain. Sulfonamides such as co-trimoxazole increase bilirubin displacement from albumin. This free bilirubin can readily cross the neonatal BBB and cause life-threatening kernicterus. Although penicillins and cephalosporins can cross the BBB more readily in neonates, gentamicin cannot.

6. Half-life of drugs

Answer: All false

In each half-life the amount of drug excreted decreases. Steady state occurs after 4–5 half-lives. Loading doses do not decrease the time to steady state, but help to get levels into range more quickly. Steady plasma levels can only be achieved with drugs with short half-lives by giving them by continuous infusion. The half-life is the time for the drug plasma concentration to decrease from its peak level by half.

7. Neonatal hepatic metabolism

Answers: A B C

Diazepam is metabolised in the liver and this metabolism is decreased in neonates. Grey baby syndrome is a toxic effect of chloramphenicol in neonates unlike aplastic anaemia which is idiosyncratic. Glucuronidation, which is the usual pathway for paracetamol metabolism, is reduced in neonates. Instead of this, however, neonates sulfate paracetamol very efficiently. Theophylline could be used effectively in neonates. However, caffeine is less toxic, has a much longer half-life, and is a large active metabolite of theophylline in neonates and thus is the preferred agent for apnoea. Gentamicin is renally cleared in all age groups.

8. Severe renal failure

Answers: A E

Digoxin is renally cleared and thus doses must decrease in renal failure. Cephalosporins and penicillins are both cerebral irritants and should both be used with caution in severe renal failure. Sucralfate contains aluminium which is absorbed and will accumulate over the long term in severe renal failure, to produce encephalopathy. Aminoglycosides should be given based on the drug levels and not on a routine basis particularly when there is renal impairment. Haemodialysis is more effective than peritoneal dialysis at reducing levels of low-molecular-weight drugs, drugs with low protein binding, water-soluble drugs and drugs with a low volume of distribution.

9. Systemic lupus erythematosus

Answers: A C D E

Slow acetylators are predisposed to spontaneous and drug-induced systemic lupus erythematosus (SLE). Although slow acetylators, who have a reduced metabolism of isoniazid, are more prone to developing SLE, they may be unaffected. Many drugs such as phenytoin, penicillin, clonidine, methyldopa, beta-blockers and sulfonamides may induce SLE.

10. Impaired liver function

Answers: B C E

Morphine is metabolised in the liver and renally cleared. Impaired liver function causes opiate accumulation and central nervous system depression, thereby causing respiratory depression. Hypokalaemia is a serious problem with the use of loop and thiazide diuretics particularly in liver impairment. Clotting factors are reduced in liver impairment, thus increasing the chances of bleeding in children on warfarin. Cyclosporin causes renal toxicity but is hepatically metabolised, thus necessitating a reduced dose in liver impairment. Liver impairment may lead to hypoproteinaemia. This will lead to less protein binding of highly protein-bound drugs such as phenytoin. The extra free (active) phenytoin will increase the chances of toxicity even if the overall amount of plasma phenytoin remains the same.

11. Therapeutic drug monitoring

Answers: A C

Very high vancomycin levels may lead to toxic effects, such as renal impairment. Low levels render the drug ineffective. It is acceptable for Gentamicin levels to be unrecordable before the next dose, due to the post-antibiotic effect of bacteria stasis. Low potassium levels make cells more sensitive to digoxin, and toxicity is more likely to be seen even within the therapeutic range. Phenytoin levels do not reach steady-state levels for about a week and any levels taken before this will simply show a snapshot of the level which will keep changing. Carbamazepine induces auto-induction and thus levels tend to drop off after about 2 weeks.

12. Ingestion of iron

Answer: D

The clinical features of iron overdose are divided into three stages. The first stage occurs within a few hours and is characterized by nausea, vomiting, abdominal pain, and haematemesis. The second stage, 8–16 hours after ingestion is when there is apparent recovery and the patient may be asymptomatic. In the third stage, 16–20 hours after ingestion, hypoglycaemia and metabolic acidosis usually develop. Hepatic failure takes 2–4 days after ingestion to manifest. Toxicity is unlikely to occur if < 20 mg/kg of elemental iron was ingested, while toxicity may occur if this level was > 20 mg/kg. Significant iron poisoning is likely to ensue after 60 mg/kg has been ingested. The iron chelating agent, desferrioxamine, is effective in limiting toxicity. It is usually administered orally but in cases of severe toxicity (> 60 mg/kg) desferrioxamine should be given intravenously. An abdominal X-ray is of use because elemental iron is radio-opaque, and therefore is helpful for documenting which part of the gastrointestinal tract the iron is in. If it is only in the stomach, a gastric lavage is indicated, but if it is in the intestine, oral desferrioxamine is the treatment of choice, together with a bowel stimulant.

13. Toxic substance ingestion/inhalation

Answers: A B E

Acute salicylate ingestion can cause a metabolic alkalosis initially, with a metabolic acidosis normally ensuing thereafter. Induced emesis is definitely contraindicated when a corrosive substance is ingested, to limit further mucosal damage. Chronic lead poisoning leads to the behavioural and cognitive disturbances seen in these patients, but not in the acute phase. Tricyclic antidepressants cause the anticholinergic effects of urinary retention, dry mouth and pupillary dilatation – not constriction. Carbon monoxide poisoning does cause tissue hypoxia despite a normal PaO_2.

14. B: Neonates have a higher volume of distribution for water-soluble drugs

All the answers are true for benzylpenicillin in the neonate, but the reason for the higher dose is only due to the higher volume of distribution caused by the increased extracellular fluid.

15. C: Decreased albumin levels lead to increased 'free' phenytoin

The main reason for the lower plasma phenytoin levels is that of the decreased albumin levels. The phenytoin excretion is reasonable from birth. Albumin binding is not as tight as it is in children, but bilirubin rarely plays a part in displacing large amounts unless levels are very high. The overall plasma concentration of phenytoin needs to be lower because there is more free (non-bound) drug and thus dosing can be reduced as compared to adults and children.

16. B: Neonatal livers are unable to glucuronidate high doses of chloramphenicol

Glucuronidation is one of the last metabolic processes to be established in neonates. Some drugs are sulphated in preference, but chloramphenicol is not. Thus high doses of chloramphenicol are not able to be metabolised, and toxic levels go into the central nervous system and other organs, to produce the often fatal effects of the grey baby syndrome.

17. C: Increase the dose by about 20% and monitor the child

Phenytoin demonstrates saturable kinetics within the therapeutic range. This means that large dose adjustments just outside the range (10–20 mg/L) or within the range are likely to lead to very large variations in plasma levels and likely to send the child toxic. Although the levels are likely to increase a little over the next few days until steady state is reached, this is unlikely to be adequate or fast enough for this patient. Albumin may well be affecting the level, but the patient needs to be treated now, irrespective of the amount of free phenytoin. Doubling or re-loading the patient should only be considered in an emergency.

18. E: Administer activated charcoal

The most appropriate management in this instance would be to administer activated charcoal, to limit further absorption of paracetamol. Induced emesis with ipecacuanha is now generally contraindicated. Plasma paracetamol levels are only useful after 4 hours of ingestion. A gastric lavage may be beneficial, but when you are given these five choices it would not be the first choice of treatment. N-Acetylcysteine would not be the first line of treatment either.

19. NEONATAL PHARMACOKINETICS

1. G – Volume of distribution
Neonates have a far greater relative extracellular fluid volume than infants (who have a far greater relative fat content) thus neonates require relatively more water soluble drug to achieve the same plasma concentration.

2. F – Protein binding
Neonates generally have lower protein concentrations and reduced protein-building capacity. This leads to increased "free" phenytoin, which is able to act on receptors.

3. E – Renal function
Benzylpenicillin is renally cleared. Neonates have a reduced renal clearance and they do not require such frequent dosing despite requiring the same doses (if not higher) on a mg/kg basis.

20. THERAPEUTIC DRUG MONITORING

1. B – Carbamazepine
Carbamazepine plasma concentrations will increase over the first couple of weeks of treatment. However, before steady-state is reached carbamazepine induces its own metabolism leading to increased rates of metabolism and reduction of plasma levels.

2. A – Phenytoin
Phenytoin has saturable kinetics when plasma levels are in (or close to) the therapeutic range. Thus dose increases must be small if plasma levels are close to the therapeutic range to avoid a huge increase in plasma levels and the onset of toxicity.

3.   D – Digoxin

Digoxin preparations have different bioavailabilities. The liquid has greater bioavailability than the tablets and thus less liquid is required (in terms of mg of digoxin) than tablets, to achieve the same plasma concentration.

Dermatology

Helen Goodyear

Multiple Choice Questions

1. Alopecia is a recognised feature of
- ○ A Pachyonychia congenita
- ○ B Chédiak–Higashi syndrome
- ○ C Cyclosporin therapy
- ○ D Hartnup disease
- ○ E Incontinentia pigmenti

2. The following is true of systemic lupus erythematosus (SLE)
- ○ A non-scarring alopecia is a typical feature
- ○ B neonatal lupus is associated with transient heart block
- ○ C Gottron papules are a typical feature
- ○ D an erythematous malar rash is pathognomonic
- ○ E treatment with benzylpenicillin is a recognised precipitant

3. The following is true of the structure and function of normal skin
- ○ A the epidermis has a rich blood supply
- ○ B the skin absorbs oxygen
- ○ C vitamin D_3 is synthesised in the stratum corneum
- ○ D the dermis is thicker in neonates compared to adults
- ○ E melanocytes are present in the dermis

4. A nappy rash is a recognised feature of
- ○ A acrodermatitis enteropathica
- ○ B Kawasaki disease
- ○ C scabies
- ○ D epidermolysis bullosa
- ○ E Langerhans cell histiocytosis

5. Disorders presenting as a collodion baby include

○ A ichthyosis vulgaris
○ B Gaucher disease
○ C Bloom syndrome
○ D urticaria pigmentosa
○ E Sjögren–Larsson syndrome

6. Photosensitivity is a feature of

○ A Netherton syndrome
○ B trichothiodystrophy
○ C Rothmund–Thomson syndrome
○ D Gitelman syndrome
○ E Marfan syndrome

7. In psoriasis

○ A the rash typically affects the flexor surfaces
○ B boys tend to be affected by psoriasis at a younger age than girls
○ C there is a 25% chance of getting psoriasis if a first degree relative is affected
○ D the incidence of arthropathy is higher in patients with nail changes
○ E provoking factors include penicillin therapy

8. The listed erythemas are correctly linked with their recognised causative factors

○ A herpes simplex virus and erythema marginatum
○ B oral contraceptive pill and erythema nodosum
○ C *Staphylococcus aureus* and erythema neonatorum
○ D viral infections and toxic erythemas
○ E *Borrelia burgdorferi* and erythema migrans

9. The following facts are true about viral infections

○ A perianal warts in a child under 2 years of age are most commonly acquired due to sexual abuse
○ B plantar warts are due to a poxvirus
○ C exanthem subitum is due to parvovirus B19
○ D mollusca contagiosa are more common in children with atopic eczema than in those with normal skin
○ E hand, foot and mouth disease is due to an enterovirus

10. The following is true of birthmarks

○ A sebaceous naevi characteristically develop in the first 6 months of life
○ B laser therapy is recommended for salmon patches
○ C a large melanocytic bathing trunk naevus is associated with a 50% increase in risk of melanoma formation

○ D a large port wine stain is associated with the Kasabach–Merritt syndrome

○ E strawberry naevi are more common in pre-term infants

11. Nail changes are a recognised feature of

○ A epidermolysis bullosa (EB)
○ B hypothyroidism
○ C pityriasis rubra pilaris
○ D alopecia areata
○ E atopic eczema

12. In the treatment of childhood atopic eczema

○ A Chinese herbal treatment is recommended for infants
○ B Betnovate and Dermovate are commonly used
○ C tacrolimus ointment is an effective therapy for moderate to severe eczema
○ D short courses of oral cyclosporin are used for severe eczema
○ E resistance of *Staphylococcus aureus* to erythromycin is present in around one third of cases

13. Recognised causes of neonatal erythroderma include

○ A Omenn syndrome
○ B cystic fibrosis
○ C galactosaemia
○ D multiple carboxylase deficiency
○ E Di George syndrome

14. The following is true of of acne

○ A it typically presents between the ages of 7 and 12 years
○ B vitamin A derivatives are first-line therapy
○ C it should be investigated if it appears in a child < 1 year of age
○ D cyproterone acetate is an effective treatment for boys
○ E it is a recognised feature of Cushing syndrome

15. Ichthyosis due to steroid sulphatase deficiency

○ A affects girls
○ B is associated with pyloric stenosis
○ C has an incidence of 1 in 250
○ D is characterised by fine light scaling
○ E has prolonged labour as a recognised feature

Best of Five Questions

16. **A 2-year-old girl has been affected since she was 6 months of age by an itchy red rash of the limb flexures which comes and goes. Which would be the MOST suitable initial treatment?**

- ○ A Diet free from cow's milk
- ○ B Betnovate cream applied twice daily
- ○ C Use of regular emollient therapy
- ○ D Chinese herbal therapy
- ○ E Tacrolimus 0.03% ointment

17. **An 8-year-old girl has severe generalised atopic eczema and has attended clinic monthly for the last 6 months. She has missed nearly 4 weeks of school in the last 2 months. Which treatment would be MOST appropriate?**

- ○ A Twice-daily application of emollient wet wraps
- ○ B Twice-daily application of Eumovate cream
- ○ C Oral acitretin
- ○ D Oral cyclosporin
- ○ E Twice daily application of Dermovate cream

18. **A 9-month-old boy has had a red rash affecting his trunk and limbs for the last 3 months which you diagnose as scabies. Which of the following is MOST likely?**

- ○ A Mild itchiness
- ○ B Other family members are unaffected
- ○ C There are no lesions on the face
- ○ D Peeling of skin on the palms and soles
- ○ E Persistent nodules after treatment

19. **A 1-month-old boy presents to the casualty department with a high temperature and widespread erythematous skin with peeling skin on the fingers and soles of the feet. Of the following information, which are you MOST likely to include in your advice to parents?**

- ○ A Topical fucidin ointment is the treatment of choice
- ○ B There is skin infection due to *Staphylococcus epidermidis*
- ○ C This is a common infantile presentation of psoriasis
- ○ D An intravenous cannula will need to be sited
- ○ E Scabies is the underlying cause

20. **A 9-year-old girl has had widespread plaque psoriasis for the last 3 years affecting her limbs, trunk and face. Many treatments have been tried without success. She has missed several weeks of school and has regularly attended the dermatology clinic. Which of the following therapies is the MOST appropriate?**

- A Psoralen ultraviolet A (PUVA)
- B Vitamin D analogues
- C Betnovate 1 in 4 cream
- D Methotrexate
- E Penicillin V

21. **A 6-year-old girl complains of a red scaly rash on the limbs. On examination, you find numerous plaques affecting the arms and legs. Which of the following is MOST likely?**

- A Onset of rash was in the first 2 years of life
- B Rubbing the skin provokes white scaling
- C Oral lesions with a white reticulate surface
- D Flexural sites are affected
- E Severe destructive arthritis which symmetrically affects large joints

22. **An 18-month-old boy is referred by his GP with a 5-day history of not eating and drinking, being unwell, and having multiple mouth and lip ulcers and white lesions on the tongue. This is his first attendance at the surgery due to illness. On examination he has a pulse rate of 120 beats per minute, a blood pressure of 85/55 and his capillary refill time is less than 2 seconds. Which of the following is MOST important for his care?**

- A Oral nystatin
- B Regular mouth care including antiseptic mouth washes
- C Intravenous aciclovir
- D Intravenous fluids
- E Oral paracetamol

23. **The parents of a 2-year-old girl with moderately severe eczema affecting mainly her trunk, face and limb flexures ask for advice on the condition. Which of the following recommendations is MOST applicable?**

- A She should not be taken swimming
- B Betnovate cream should be applied for her facial eczema
- C Dithranol in Lassar's paste should be applied twice daily to the limbs
- D They should join their local FIRST support group
- E They should keep her bedroom at a constant temperature

24. A child with atopic eczema presents with a flare-up of the eczema. You would suspect herpes simplex virus (HSV) rather than bacterial infection if which ONE of the following occurred?

  ○ A The lesions affected the face

  ○ B There were constitutional symptoms such as vomiting, diarrhoea and pyrexia

  ○ C Lesions were present at different stages

  ○ D Extensor sites were affected

  ○ E Pustules were present

25. A 13-month-old boy has an itchy red rash and coryzal symptoms. Which one of the following is MOST likely?

  ○ A The pattern of rash is usually helpful in making the diagnosis

  ○ B The rash will have resolved within a week

  ○ C An urticarial rash rarely occurs with viral infections

  ○ D The season may give a clue to the diagnosis

  ○ E Investigating the cause of the rash does not affect management

26. You are writing a departmental advice sheet on scabies. Which is the MOST appropriate recommendation for the treatment period?

  ○ A Wash all clothes, towels and bed-linen at the start of treatment

  ○ B Apply treatment only from the neck downwards

  ○ C Reapply treatment each time the hands are washed

  ○ D Use a benzyl benzoate lotion

  ○ E Use an alcohol-based preparation

27. An 8-year-old girl presents with a 1-day history of urticarial rash. In your advice to the girl and her parents, what would you be MOST likely to say?

  ○ A The rash may be due to a viral infection

  ○ B Individual lesions tend to last for > 24 hours and then resolve

  ○ C Cool bedroom temperatures help to improve symptoms

  ○ D Aspirin helps symptoms

  ○ E A causal agent is identified in 90% of cases

Extended Matching Questions

28. Theme: Photosensitive rashes

A   Neonatal lupus erythematosus
B   Juvenile spring eruption
C   Hartnup disease
D   Xeroderma pigmentosa
E   Congenital erythropoietic protoporphyria
F   Rothmund–Thomson syndrome
G   Bloom syndrome
H   Cockayne syndrome

For each child described below with a photosensitive rash, select the MOST likely condition from the above list. Each option may be used once, more than once, or not at all.

  ○   1. A 3-month-old girl presents with erythematous scaly lesions on the face after being outside in the sunlight. Physical examination is otherwise unremarkable.

  ○   2. A 5-year-old boy whose parents are first cousins presents with a history of erythema and telangiectasia on his face, and the dorsa of the hands and forearms. His mother is concerned about this because her brother died in this late-30s with leukaemia. Physical examination shows his height and weight to be less than the third centile, and well-demarcated areas of hypopigmentation and hyperpigmentation on his trunk.

  ○   3. A 5-year-old boy has recently failed a hearing test for school entry. Examination shows his height and weight to be below the third centile, as well as cataracts and dental caries, and he has difficulty walking.

29. Theme: Blistering disorders

A   Herpes simplex virus infection
B   Dermatitis herpetiformis
C   Erythema multiforme
D   Epidermolysis bullosa
E   Chronic bullous disease of childhood
F   Hand, foot and mouth disease
G   Pompholyx
H   Pemphigus foliaceus

For each child described below with a blistering disorder, select the MOST likely condition from the list above. Each option may be used once, more than once, or not at all.

  ○   1. A 4-year-old boy presents with a 1-week history of tense blisters in groups on the abdomen and buttocks. He has a normal diet and has no past medical history of note. Physical examination shows lesions in the mouth, no fever, and no other abnormalities.

○   2. An 11-year-old girl presents with a 3-day history of tense clear vesicles in a bilateral distribution affecting the sides of her toes and soles of the feet. She has had three previous episodes. She had mild flexural eczema until she was 3 years of age. Physical examination is otherwise normal and she is apyrexial.

○   3. A 14-month-old boy presents with a history of tense small blisters on the hands and feet for the last 2 months. Physical examination shows no other abnormalities. He is noted to be developing normally.

30. Theme: Vesiculopustular lesions

A   Impetigo
B   Transient neonatal pustulosis
C   Scabies
D   Erythema toxicum neonatorum
E   Urticaria pigmentosa
F   Epidermolysis bullosa
G   Infantile acropustulosis
H   Incontinentia pigmenti

For each infant described below with a vesiculopustular rash, select the condition that is MOST likely from the above list. Each option may be used once, more than once, or not at all.

○   1. A 1-week-old girl is noticed to have vesicular lesions which spare her face. Examination shows that she is apyrexial, and the lesions follow Blaschko's lines and are in a linear distribution on the limbs and arranged circumferentially on the trunk.

○   2. An 8-month-old girl presents with a 6-month history of crops of itchy small vesicopustules on the hands and feet recurring at monthly intervals.

○   3. A West Indian girl baby is noticed to have vesicopustules at birth, some of which have burst to leave a pigmented macule.

answers

1. Alopecia

Answers: A E

Loss of hair (alopecia) may be present in many dermatological conditions and along with nails and mucous membranes the hair should always be inspected as part of evaluation of that condition. Pachyonychia congenita is characterised by discoloration of the nails and nail thickening which begins within the first month of life. There are different subtypes, of which one is associated with hair anomalies including alopecia. Chédiak–Higashi syndrome is incomplete occulocutaneous albinism. Characteristically there is a silvery sheen to the hair and partial albinism when compared to other family members, but not alopecia. Cyclosporin therapy causes hypertrichosis. Hartnup disease is not associated with hair loss. Many children are asymptomatic and usually the first sign is a pellagra-like rash. Hair abnormalities are common in incontinentia pigmenti. The hair is often sparse in early childhood and wiry and coarse when older. Alopecia may occur if blistering/verrucous lesions are present in the scalp, especially the vertex.

2. Systemic lupus erythematosus

Answer: E

Systemic lupus erythematosus (SLE) typically causes scarring alopecia. Heart block in neonatal lupus is permanent and not transient. Gottron papules over the knuckles and knees are present in dermatomyositis. An erythematous malar rash in a butterfly distribution is classical but is not pathognomonic as it may be present in other skin disorders. There are many drugs which may induce SLE in children who are slow acetylators and penicillin is one of them.

3. Normal skin

Answer: B

The top layer of the skin is the epidermis. It is separated from the lower layer, the dermis, by the dermoepidermal junction. The dermis has a rich blood supply, unlike the epidermis. One of the skin's functions is to absorb oxygen and excrete carbon dioxide and this accounts for 1–2% of respiration. Vitamin D_3 is synthesised in the lower layers of the epidermis (the stratum spinosum and basale) but not in the top layer of the epidermis (the stratum corneum). The dermis is less thick in neonates than in adults, collagen fibre bundles are smaller, elastin fibres are immature, vascular and neural elements are less well organised; melanocytes are present in the epidermis rather than the dermis.

4. Nappy rash

Answer: All true

Although the commonest cause of nappy rash is an irritant contact dermatitis, any dermatological disorder may present as or with a nappy rash. It is important to look at a nappy rash to see if there are skin lesions elsewhere or if there are unusual features. Acrodermatitis enteropathica due to zinc deficiency presents with skin rash around the mouth and perianal area. One of the diagnostic features of Kawasaki disease is a polymorphous erythematous rash, as well as the extremity changes affecting the skin. Scabies is due to human-to-human spread of the mite. An adult with hand lesions will readily transfer infection to the nappy area, or this can occur if the child itself has hand lesions. There are different types of epidermolysis bullosa, a group of genetically determined disorders in which the skin and mucosae involved are excessively susceptible to separation from the underlying tissues and blistering following trauma. In many types of epidermolysis bullosa the nappy area is affected.

5. Collodion baby

Answers: A B E

Collodion baby is the name given to babies who are enclosed in a shiny tight yellow film at birth. These babies tend to have an underlying ichthyosis although 10% are said to have normal skin. Icthyosis vulgaris affects the skin only with fine light scaling and is an autosomal dominant condition which affects 1 in 250 people. One of the features of Gaucher disease is ichthyosis and hence children with this condition may present at birth as collodion babies. Bloom syndrome is one of the genetic causes of photosensitivity and does not present as a collodion baby. Urticaria pigmentosa presents commonly in the first year of life as multiple yellow or red-brown macules or plaques which urticate when rubbed. In Sjögren–Larsson syndrome there is congenital ichthyosis associated with a spastic diplegia or tetraplegia and mental retardation.

6. Photosensitivity

Answers: B C

In Netherton syndrome photosensitivity is not a feature. Infants and children have a generalised exfoliative erythroderma. Trichothiodystrophy syndromes have disorders of keratinisation. PIBIDS is one of these syndromes in which the P stands for photosensitivity. Rothmund–Thomson syndrome is an autosomal recessive disorder which includes photosensitivity. Gitelman syndrome is a variant of Bartter syndrome which affects the distal tubule of the kidney and is not associated with photosensitivity. Marfan syndrome is also not associated with photosensitivity.

7. Psoriasis

Answer: D

In contrast to atopic eczema, psoriasis typically affects the extensor surfaces. Flexural sites may however be affected particularly the intertriginous areas. The age of onset tends to be younger in girls at 5–9 years and later in boys at 15–19 years. The risk of psoriasis is only 10% if a first-degree relative is affected, rising to 50% if one sibling and both parents are affected. The incidence of arthropathy is higher in psoriatic patients with nail changes, particularly pitting. However, in children with arthritis alone and no skin lesions the presence of nail pitting is not a prognostic sign for the appearance of cutaneous psoriasis. Penicillin is useful in the treatment of psoriasis. Most commonly, guttate psoriasis is associated with streptococcal infections, usually streptococcal pharyngitis, but chronic plaque psoriasis may also be associated with streptococcal infections.

8. Erythema causes

Answers: B D E

Erythema marginatum is an annular migratory erythema found in 10% of cases of rheumatic fever. Herpes simplex virus is the commonest cause of erythema multiforme. The causes of erythema nodosum are multiple, and the oral contraceptive pill and sulfonamides are causative drugs. Erythema neonatorum occurs in around 50% of neonates usually in the first 2 weeks of life. Skin lesions range from erythema to urticarial papules and pustules which contain eosinophils and are sterile. Viral infections are the most common cause of toxic erythemas (erythema accompanied with a fever and systemic symptoms). Erythema migrans occurs in Lyme disease, which is caused by the spirochete *Borrelia burgdorferi* and transmitted by *Ixodes* ticks. There is a red papule at the site of the tick bite which expands to form a large annular erythematous lesion.

9. Viral infections

Answers: D E

Sexual abuse as the mode of transmission of perianal warts is more of concern in children over the age of 2 years. Children may acquire perianal warts in a number of ways and vertical transmission from the mother's genital tract, either prenatally or during delivery, is the likeliest mode of spread if warts are present at birth or during the first 2 years. Inoculation of the virus from hand lesions present on the hands of the child or the carer's hands is another common cause. Non-sexual transmission may also occur by innocent contact due to sharing baths or towels with infected adults. Warts are due to human papillomavirus. The lesions of mollusca contagiosa, known as water warts, are due to a poxvirus. Exanthem subitum, also know as roseola infantum, is due to human herpes virus type 6 or type 7. Erythema infectiosum, know as slapped cheek or fifth disease, is due to parvovirus B19 infection.

10. Birthmarks

Answer: E

Sebaceous naevi are characteristically present at birth. Salmon patches or stork bites do not need any treatment. Those on the face typically resolve spontaneously while those on the neck persist in 10–20% of cases but tend to be hidden by hair. Laser therapy is used to treat port wine stains that are of cosmetic concern. Giant melanocytic naevi do carry an increased risk of melanoma but this is not as high as 50% and recent studies quote incidences between 4% and 14%. Port wine stains are associated with Sturge–Weber syndrome and Klippel–Trenaunay–Weber syndrome; Kasabach–Merritt syndrome is due to a rapidly enlarging strawberry haemangioma. Strawberry naevi are more common in pre-term infants.

11. Nail changes

Answer: All true

EB is the name given to a group of genetically determined disorders in which the skin and mucosae are excessively susceptible to separation from the underlying tissues and blistering following trauma. Nails may be affected in both junctional and dystrophic EB. In hypothyroidism there is decreased nail growth, ridging, and brittleness. Pityriasis rubra pilaris is an erythematous eruption of unknown aetiology characterised by palmoplantar keratoderma (thickening of skin on palms and soles). There are different types with nail features including thickened curved nails and terminal hyperaemia (half-and-half nail). Nail changes in alopecia areata are usually in the form of nail pitting. Such changes tend to be greater in those with more severe disease. In atopic eczema there may be nail pitting, Beau's lines and onycholysis (separation of the nail plate from the nail bed).

12. Childhood atopic eczema

Answers: C D

Chinese herbal treatment is not usually recommended for children less than 2 years of age. Children require monitoring of liver and renal function and the herbal treatment should be discontinued if these tests become deranged. Betnovate is a potent topical steroid and Dermovate is a very potent topical steroid which would only be used in specialist centres when atopic eczema is not responding to use of less potent topical steroid creams and other measures. Topical tacrolimus (Protopic) is a relative new treatment for moderate-to-severe atopic eczema. If eczema is unresponsive to topical therapy, including bandaging techniques, then systemic therapy is used: either oral prednisolone or cyclosporin may be given in short courses of 3–6 months. Resistance to erythromycin by *Staphylococcus aureus* is one of the reasons that eczema fails to improve after a course of antibiotics, but resistance rates are not as high as 33% and in hospital-acquired infection are probably nearer 20%.

13. Neonatal erythroderma

Answers: A B D E

In Omenn syndrome, infants are erythrodermic and have failure to thrive, a history of recurrent infections, and prominent lymphadenopathy. Cystic fibrosis can present, usually in the first 6 months of life, with a severe dermatitis which particular affects the perioral and nappy areas. There is failure to thrive. The dermatitis precedes the onset of lung and gastrointestinal symptoms. Zinc levels may be slightly low but the dermatitis does not improve with zinc therapy (unlike acrodermatitis enteropathica). Neonatal erythroderma is not a feature of galactosaemia. The neonatal form of multiple carboxylase deficiency presents in the first few weeks of life with a marked dermatitis presenting on the face and spreading to the perianal and flexural areas. Di George syndrome has been reported as causing a widespread eczematous dermatitis.

14. Acne

Answer: E

Acne typically presents between the ages of 10 and 16 years. Vitamin A derivatives (isotretinoin) are used for severe acne which does not respond to other therapies. Neonatal and infantile acne are relatively common and (providing there are no other concerns) do not need investigation. Acne appearing for the first time between the ages of 1 and 7 years should always be investigated. Cyproterone acetate with ethinylestradiol (Dianette) is used for treatment of acne in girls. Causes of hyperandrogenism including Cushing disease should be thought of in young girls with acne (aged 1-7 years).

15. Ichthyosis due to steroid sulphatase deficiency

Answers: B E

Ichthyosis due to steroid sulphatase deficiency is X-linked and therefore is found in boys. It can be associated with pyloric stenosis. Ichthyosis vulgaris is the most common inherited ichthyosis and has an incidence of 1 in 250. X-linked steroid sulphatase deficiency is the next most common with an incidence of 1 in 2000. Scaling is dark brown in contrast to the fine light scaling of ichthyosis vulgaris. There is prolonged labour due to placental sulphatase deficiency.

16. C: Use of regular emollient therapy

This is atopic eczema. It is the initial treatment which is being considered and this should include use of emollients such as bath oils, soap substitutes and moisturisers. A diet free of cow's milk may be considered, especially in those less than 1 year of age, for severe atopic eczema. Betnovate cream is a potent topical steroid which is not used routinely in the treatment of childhood atopic eczema. Chinese herbal therapy has often been used but would not be an initial recommendation for mild to moderate atopic eczema. Likewise, topical tacrolimus is for children with eczema which is moderate to severe and which is not responding to treatment.

17. D: Oral cyclosporin

This is chronic atopic eczema that is not responding to treatment because she is coming to clinic monthly and is taking a lot of time off school. A short course of oral cyclosporin is one of the systemic therapies used for atopic eczema not responding to topical therapies. Emollient wet wraps may help as part of the treatment regimen, but other therapy is needed and wet wraps are often not well tolerated by older children. Eumovate cream is a moderately potent topical steroid cream which would already have been used in this case. Acitretin is used in the treatment of psoriasis and ichthyotic disorders. Dermovate cream is a potent topical steroid cream. Potent steroid creams should be used cautiously in children due to local skin side-effects and, as the eczema is generalised, there should be concern about the child developing Cushing syndrome.

18. E: Persistent nodules after treatment

Scabetic nodules are a reaction to the mite and often persist after successful treatment for up to 3 months. Scabies is an intensely itchy skin eruption and it is highly likely that the parents, at least, will be affected as they will be regularly in contact with his skin while dressing or bathing him, and during nappy changes. Infants with scabies quite often get lesions on the head and face. Peeling of skin on the palms and soles may occur after scabies especially if secondary bacterial infection occurs, although this is not a typical feature.

19. D: An intravenous cannula will need to be sited

This is staphylococcal scalded skin syndrome. Systemic antibiotics are needed. Use of topical fucidin should be restricted as resistant staphylococci emerge. The skin infection is due to toxin-producing *Staphylococcus aureus* and not *Staphylococcus epidermidis*. Psoriasis in infancy is not common and presents with typical psoriatic patches rather than in the manner described in the question. Scabies tends to have an incubation period of about 1 month and would only present in this way if there was a secondary bacterial infection.

20. D: Methotrexate

This is chronic plaque psoriasis which is relapsing often, and which is not under control. Many topical therapies will have been used over a 3-year period. Systemic therapy is warranted and methotrexate is one of the systemic drugs used for psoriasis. PUVA involves the use of phytotoxic psoralens in combination with ultraviolet A light and tends not to be used in children (particularly in those younger than teenagers) because its use increases the risk of skin cancer. Vitamin D analogues (eg Dovonex) are used for mild to moderate psoriasis when < 40% of the skin area is affected. Penicillin V is used in the treatment of guttate psoriasis which may be triggered by streptococcal infection and in other forms of psoriasis only if there is evidence of streptococcal infection.

21. B: Rubbing the skin provokes white scaling

This is chronic plaque psoriasis. If erythematous plaques are present and are due to psoriasis then rubbing produces the typical white scale. Less than 2% of psoriasis presents in the first 2 years of life and 10% of cases will have an onset age of under 10 years. Girls tend to be affected between the ages of 5 and 9 years and boys between 15 and 19 years. Lesions in the mouth affecting the buccal mucosa with a white reticulate surface are typical of lichen planus. Psoriasis tends to affect the extensor surfaces. Psoriatic arthritis is occasionally severely destructive. It tends to be an asymmetrical arthritis.

22. E: Oral paracetamol

This is primary herpes simplex gingivostomatitis. Pain relief is needed and paracetamol is appropriate. The tongue is often white and this is not usually due to *Candida*. Mouth care is difficult to perform in children, and most mouth washes sting causing further misery to the child. Aciclovir stops further viral replication but does not help when there are multiple lesions present. Some children treated with aciclovir develop poorer antibody responses. This child is highly unlikely to be immunocompromised or to have skin disease as it is his first attendance at the GP surgery. Intravenous fluids may be needed in very severe cases but children often start to drink after adequate analgesia has been given.

23. E: They should keep her bedroom at a constant temperature

Atopic eczema can be exacerbated by changes in temperature, particularly in conditions of overheating. The eczema is of mild-to-moderate severity and treatment would not be classed as successful if she was unable to go swimming. Betnovate cream is a potent topical steroid cream and is not used to treat facial eczema in children. Dithranol in Lassar's paste is a treatment for psoriasis, and the FIRST support group is actually for ichthyosis.

24. C: Lesions were present at different stages

This is eczema herpeticum. Lesions may affect the face and constitutional symptoms may be present with both bacterial and HSV infection. Lesions present at different stages is one of the features of HSV infection. Severe eczema may affect extensor surfaces and both bacterial and HSV infection are associated with flare-up of the eczema. Pustules may be present in both conditions.

25. D: The season may give a clue to the diagnosis

Some infections are more common in certain seasons, for example enteroviruses are more common in summer and autumn. The pattern of rash may be helpful in making a diagnosis (as in hand, foot and mouth disease) but is often non-specific in the majority of cases of viral rash. Rashes associated with viral infections may last for 2–3 weeks and sometimes longer. Urticarial rashes occur quite often with viral infections. If the cause of the rash is found to be a viral infection which may affect the fetus (eg rubella) or immunocompromised patients (eg chickenpox) then those who might come into contact with the patient will be offered advice and treatment as appropriate.

26. C: Reapply treatment each time the hands are washed

When treating scabies the lotion must be reapplied every time the hands are washed. If not, this is a common cause of treatment failure. Clothes, towels and bed-linen should be washed at the end of treatment. If there are lesions on the head then treatment will not be successful unless the lotion is applied to these lesions. Benzyl benzoate is not recommended for treatment of children because it is an irritant and is less effective than malathion-based treatments. Alcohol-based preparations tend to sting and are therefore not recommended for use in children.

27. A: The rash may be due to a viral infection

Viral infections are a common cause of urticarial rashes. Individual lesions typically are short-lived and last less than 24 hours. Urticaria can be due to or can be made worse by cold temperatures. Salicylic acid is a cause of urticaria. About 50% of cases of urticaria are idiopathic.

28. PHOTOSENSITIVE RASHES

1.   A – Neonatal lupus erythematosus
Neonatal lupus erythematosus (NLE) may be present at birth but can develop a number of weeks later. It can be induced by UV light and there have been a few reports of NLE after phototherapy for hyperbilirubinaemia.

2.   G – Bloom syndrome
Bloom syndrome is an autosomal recessive condition characterised by growth retardation, photosensitivity, pigment abnormalities, and telangiectasia. There is a cancer predisposition in Bloom syndrome which includes leukaemia and lymphomas. Poikiloderma (atrophic pigmentary telangiectasia) is characteristic of Rothmund–Thomson syndrome in which the malignancies tend to be of the skin or bone (osteosarcoma).

3.   H – Cockayne syndrome
Cockayne syndrome is an autosomal dominant condition characterised by growth failure, progressive neurological deterioration, dental caries, eye abnormalities including cataracts, and sensorineural hearing loss. Xeroderma pigmentosum is an autosomal recessive condition characterised by extreme

photosensitivity, freckling and skin malignancy in childhood. Neurological complications occur in 20%. Eye abnormalities include loss of lashes, ectropion, photophobia, conjunctival telangiectasia and corneal abnormalities.

29. BLISTERING DISORDERS

1. E – Chronic bullous disease of childhood

Chronic bullous disease of childhood is also known as linear immunoglobulin A disease. It typically presents in children aged over 3 years with tense small (1–3 mm) blisters on an erythematous background. Lesions characteristically affect the perianal area and spread to the trunk, thighs, limbs, hands and feet. There may be mucosal involvement of the mouth, the genitals, and eyes and nose. Lesions usually appear abruptly but may present as a pruritic rash over a number of weeks. Dermatitis herpetiformis tends to present later than chronic bullous disease of childhood and affects symmetrically the elbows, knees and buttocks. Mouth involvement is rare. Herpes simplex virus infection would usually be a primary one with mouth and other sites of the body affected and the child would be expected to have constitutional symptoms including fever. Pemphigus is very rare in childhood and tends to occur in adults in middle age. In pemphigus foliaceus, mucous membranes are rarely affected and mouth lesions are atypical. In erythema multiforme the lesions are symmetrical red papules, some of which form target lesions and blister. Mouth lesions may be present.

2. G – Pompholyx

Pompholyx is rare in children aged less than 10 years. It is characterised by sudden onset of crops of clear vesicles and is usually bilateral, affecting the sides of fingers and toes, palms and soles. A history of previous episodes is common. It is commonly found in children who have a personal or family history of atopy. Hand, foot and mouth disease is characterised by lesions on the hands and in the mouth, as well as on the feet, and it is not usually recurrent. Dermatitis herpetiformis can involve the palms and soles but usually affects the flexural aspects of digits rather than the sides and would also usually be found on other sites of the body.

3. D – Epidermolysis bullosa

Epidermolysis bullosa simplex is localised to friction sites, usually the hands and feet, and typically has its onset in early childhood around the time the child begins to crawl or walk.

30. VESICULOPUSTULAR LESIONS

1. H – Incontinentia pigmenti

Incontinentia pigmenti is an X-linked dominant condition and is usually lethal in boys. Lesions typically develop in the first week of life and the first stage is a vesicular one. If widespread impetigo was present, the baby would be expected to have systemic symptoms including pyrexia. It is rather early for a

answers

scabies rash to develop and this does not follow Blaschko's lines. Lesions are papules as well as vesicles. Erythema toxicum neonatorum does not follow Blaschko's lines. Epidermolysis bullosa often presents at birth with absence of skin.

2.   G – Infantile acropustulosis

Infantile acropustulosis usually presents in the first few months of life and is characterised by recurrent crops of vesicopustules on the hands and feet.

3.   B – Transient neonatal pustulosis

Transient neonatal pustulosis is characterised by pustules present at birth, some of which may have ruptured. They leave a pigmented macule which may persist for up to 3 months. It is more common in black skin.

Urticaria pigmentosa commonly presents in the first year of life but may be present at birth. These are skin-coloured or red brown macules which urticate when rubbed.

Endocrinology

Fiona Regan and Heather Mitchell

Multiple Choice Questions

1. The following is true of type 1 diabetes mellitus in children aged 0–14 years

- ○ A the highest worldwide incidence is in Finland
- ○ B there is a family history of type 1 diabetes in 5% of newly diagnosed children
- ○ C the risk for an offspring is higher if the mother rather than the father has type 1 diabetes mellitus
- ○ D glutamic acid decarboxylase antibodies are commonly found at diagnosis
- ○ E there is an increased incidence of cystic fibrosis

2. The following are syndromes of G protein abnormalities

- ○ A vitamin D-dependent rickets
- ○ B De Morsier syndrome
- ○ C McCune–Albright syndrome
- ○ D nephrogenic diabetes insipidus
- ○ E pseudohypoparathyroidism

3. The following statements are true about gonadotrophins

- ○ A in males, Leydig cells respond to follicle-stimulating hormone (FSH)
- ○ B excretion of FSH and luteinising hormone are inhibited by inhibin
- ○ C gonadotrophins decline during early childhood
- ○ D in females, FSH binds to glomerulosa cells
- ○ E synthesis and excretion of FSH and LH are stimulated by gonadotrophin-releasing hormone

4. The following hormones are secreted from the pituitary gland

- ○ A gonadotrophin-releasing hormone
- ○ B prolactin
- ○ C vasopressin
- ○ D growth hormone
- ○ E thyroid-stimulating hormone

questions

5. Concerning physiological progression of puberty

- A in girls pubic hair appears prior to the onset of breast development
- B up to 75% of boys will develop an element of gynaecomastia
- C peak height velocity in boys coincides with genital stage 2
- D menarche indicates cessation of growth in girls
- E follicle-stimulating hormone (FSH) in boys stimulates testosterone production

6. The following statements are true of septo-optic dysplasia

- A it is a developmental abnormality of the mid-line structures of the brain
- B the pituitary deficiencies may progress
- C optic nerve hypoplasia is present
- D there is absence of the septum pellucidum
- E the most common hormone deficiency is of adrenocorticotrophic hormone

7. Delayed puberty

- A is more common in girls
- B in boys is usually secondary to hypogonadotrophic hypogonadism
- C in Klinefelter syndrome is usually associated with anosmia
- D in ovarian failure investigations demonstrate a low LH and FSH
- E in boys is best treated with oral testosterone

8. The following are tests for growth hormone insufficiency

- A sleep deprivation
- B clonidine
- C oral glucose tolerance test
- D glucagon
- E insulin-induced hypoglycaemia

9. Which of the following are licensed indications for treatment with growth hormone

- A growth hormone deficiency
- B small for gestational age
- C chronic renal failure
- D Prader–Willi syndrome
- E achondroplasia

10. It is true that hyperthyroidism

- A in the neonate can occur in infants of mothers with both active and inactive hyperthyroidism
- B in childhood secondary to Graves disease is not usually associated with a thyroid goitre
- C may result in polyuria and nocturia

○ D commonly has an acute onset in childhood
○ E that is treated medically will result in long-term remission in 50% of children within 2 years

11. The following is true about growth

○ A insulin-like growth factor(IGF)-2 influences intra-uterine growth
○ B nutrition affects the childhood phase of growth
○ C maternal blood pressure affects intra-uterine growth
○ D growth hormone affects growth from birth to puberty
○ E sex hormones influence the pubertal growth spurt.

12. Cushing's syndrome

○ A in childhood is usually secondary to pituitary tumours
○ B commonly results in obese tall children
○ C is normally straightforward to diagnose in childhood
○ D when secondary to Cushing's disease has been caused by adrenal pathology
○ E that is associated with a low ACTH and failure to suppress cortisol with high-dose dexamethasone is likely to be due to an adrenal tumour

13. The following are features of achondroplasia

○ A mid-facial hypoplasia
○ B prominent forehead
○ C hydrocephalus
○ D short limbs and spine
○ E otitis media

14. With regard to bone metabolism

○ A the parathyroid (PTH) and calcitonin genes are located on chromosome 10
○ B in response to hypocalcaemia PTH has an immediate effect on intestinal absorption
○ C vitamin D-dependent rickets type 2 is caused by deficiency of 1α hydroxylation of 25 hydroxyvitamin D
○ D bone disease of prematurity is caused by vitamin D deficiency
○ E peak bone mass may be positively influenced by obesity

15. The following statements are true of childhood tall stature

○ A Klinefelter syndrome is associated with anosmia
○ B Marfan syndrome is associated with pneumothorax
○ C in Soto syndrome the head circumference is proportional to length
○ D it is associated with a karyotype of 45XO/46XY
○ E it is associated with congenital adrenal hyperplasia

16. The improved survival rates of childhood malignancies has increased the prevalence of late endocrine effects in survivors. It is true that

- A following radiotherapy the growth hormone axis is the most susceptible to damage
- B adrenocorticotrophic hormone (ACTH) deficiency may occur up to 10 years after treatment
- C effects on spinal growth following spinal irradiation are most commonly seen in mid-childhood
- D the ovary is more susceptible to damage from chemotherapy than the testis
- E chemotherapy, particularly with alkylating agents, frequently affects the function of Leydig cells

17. Obesity

- A associated with shortened metacarpals and metatarsals may be due to Laurence–Moon–Biedl syndrome
- B is frequently associated with raised leptin levels
- C that is not associated with underlying pathology often results in reduced bone age
- D in a child under the age of 3 years, without pathological aetiology and with non-obese parents, is highly likely to persist into adult life
- E associated with craniopharyngioma is predominantly a pre-operative problem

18. The following is true of the adrenal gland

- A renin is produced in the adrenal cortex
- B cortisol is necessary for the action of adrenaline
- C secretion of adrenal androgens varies with age
- D adrenocorticotrophic hormone produces a rise in aldosterone
- E cortisol is produced from the zona glomerulosa

19. Diabetes insipidus

- A the pituitary familial form is most commonly inherited in an autosomal recessive manner
- B that has a central aetiology is predominantly seen as an isolated finding
- C may be masked by an excess of cortisol
- D as well as SIADH (syndrome of inappropriate secretion of antidiuretic hormone) can be seen in the same patient recovering from surgical resection of a craniopharyngioma
- E that is nephrogenic in origin can be treated using diuretics

20. The following are causes of delayed puberty

- ○ A Kallman syndrome
- ○ B 5-α-reductase deficiency
- ○ C polycystic ovaries
- ○ D McCune–Albright syndrome
- ○ E gonadal dysgenesis

21. Precocious/pseudoprecocious puberty

- ○ A in McCune–Albright syndrome is gonadotrophin-independent
- ○ B secondary to congenital adrenal hyperplasia may not present until mid-childhood
- ○ C if centrally mediated can be suppressed by gonadotrophin-releasing hormone (GnRH) antagonists
- ○ D if central in origin is usually idiopathic in girls
- ○ E is more common in children born prematurely

22. The following are features of Turner syndrome

- ○ A ovarian dysgenesis
- ○ B neonatal lymphoedema
- ○ C renal cysts
- ○ D congenital hypothyroidism
- ○ E ptosis

Best of Five Questions

23. A 5-year-old girl presents with short stature. She has always been short but this has become more apparent over the last year. Her height is < 2nd centile, and her weight is 2nd centile. She is asymptomatic. She is not dysmorphic. What would the MOST useful investigation be?

   O A Thyroid function test
   O B Chromosomes
   O C Coeliac screen
   O D Full blood count
   O E C reactive protein

24. A 3-month-old boy presented with a pyrexia secondary to an upper respiratory tract infection. On admission he was found to have a low blood glucose. He had been noted to have hypoglycaemic episodes on the post-natal ward which had responded to feeding. His birth weight was 3.5 kg and over the last few months his weight had been following the 25th centile. After treatment of his hypoglycaemia, examination revealed that he was not fixing and following. There were no cataracts present but fundoscopy was difficult. He had no hepatosplenomegaly and no dysmorphic features. Initial investigations revealed that concentrations of acetoacetate, β-hydroxybutyrate and free fatty acids were within the normal range. His insulin level was undetectable. What is the MOST likely diagnosis?

   O A persistent hyper-insulinaemic hypoglycaemia of infancy
   O B septo-optic dysplasia
   O C medium chain acyl-CoA dehydrogenase (MCAD) deficiency
   O D glycogen storage disease
   O E galactosaemia

25. A 13-year-old girl presents to clinic with a 1-year history of abdominal pain. She has been finding games lessons at school very tiring, but has been managing a full day at school without any problems. Her school work has remained at the same high standard. Her mother has noticed that her shoe size has not changed over the last 2 years. On examination: weight 75th centile, height 25th centile; rounded face, not flushed; pulse 60 beats per minute, blood pressure 100/60; abdomen has palpable faeces; breast stage 3; pubic/axillary hair stage 1. What is the MOST likely diagnosis?

   O A Addison's disease
   O B Cushing syndrome

○ C Hypothyroidism
○ D Chronic fatigue syndrome
○ E Constitutional delay of growth and puberty

26. **A 15-year-old boy was reviewed at a school for moderate learning difficulties because his height was > 97th centile. On examination his weight was on the 50th centile. He had bilateral testicular volumes of 2 ml and no pubic or axillary hair. He had a mild scoliosis but no other skeletal abnormalities. His mid-parental predicted height centile was the 50th. What is the MOST likely diagnosis?**

○ A Constitutional tall stature
○ B Marfan syndrome
○ C Soto syndrome
○ D Klinefelter syndrome
○ E McCune–Albright

27. **You go to review a 2-day-old baby on the post-natal ward. Ambiguous genitalia have been noted on the baby check. On examination: the baby has a genital tubercle 1.8 cm long with a urethral opening at the distal end; the genital folds are fused midline; there are no palpable gonads. What would the NEXT best step be?**

○ A Karyotype
○ B Ultrasound scan of the pelvis
○ C 17-Hydroxyprogesterone (17-OHP)
○ D Urea and electrolytes (U&E)
○ E Androgen profile

Extended Matching Questions

28. Theme: Basic science of hormones

A   Cortisol
B   Thyroxine (or Thyroid hormone)
C   Testosterone
D   Growth hormone
E   Insulin
F   Glucagon
G   Luteinising hormone
H   Aldosterone
I   Follicle-stimulating hormone
J   Oestrogen

For each of the scenarios below, select the hormone which is most likely to act in this way. Each option may be used once, more than once, or not at all.

○   1. This hormone has a continuous pattern of secretion and is regulated by a hormone produced by the pituitary gland.

○   2. This hormone has a pulsatile pattern of secretion. It binds to the Leydig cells in the male which stimulate the first step in testosterone production.

○   3. Adrenocorticotrophic hormone (ACTH) causes a temporary rise in this hormone although the effect is not sustained. The hormone is secreted from the zona glomerulosa of the adrenal cortex.

29. Theme: Pituitary hormone testing

A   Isolated pituitary hormone deficiency
B   Multiple pituitary hormone deficiencies
C   Anterior and posterior pituitary hormone deficiencies
D   Combined hypothalamic and pituitary hormone abnormalities
E   Thyroid-stimulating hormone deficiency
F   Gonadotrophin deficiency
G   Diabetes insipidus
H   Cushing's disease
I   Hyperprolactinaemia
J   Hypothalamic dysfunction

Choose the pathology from the list above which best suits the following scenarios. Each option may be used once, more than once, or not at all.

○   1. A 4-year-old boy had a craniopharyngioma removed by surgical excision. He subsequently had progressive obesity and behaviour problems

○   2. An 11-year-old girl who had previously had craniospinal irradiation for leukaemia presented with the following data after investigation for short stature with a thyrotrophin-releasing hormone (TRH) test and an insulin tolerance test.

Time (minutes)	0	30	60	90
Glucose (mmol/L)	4.2	2.4	5.0	4.8
Growth hormone (mU/L)	1	1.5	1.5	1.6
Cortisol (nmol/L)	200	220	205	205
Thyroid-stimulating hormone (mmol/L)	3	11.6	30	

○ 3. A 14-year-old boy presented with short stature associated with a bone age of 10 years. He had no pubic or axillary hair and his testicular volumes were 4 ml. He had previously been diagnosed as having anosmia.

30. Theme: Hypoglycaemia

A   Hyper-insulinaemic hypoglycaemia
B   Glycogen storage disease
C   Fatty acid oxidation defect
D   Galactosaemia
E   Growth hormone deficiency
F   Septo-optic dysplasia
G   Congenital adrenal hypoplasia
H   Congenital adrenal hyperplasia
I   Beckwith–Wiedemann syndrome
J   Infant of a diabetic mother

For each scenario described below, give the most likely cause of the hypoglycaemia from the list above. Each option may be used once, more than once, or not at all.

○ 1. A 6-week-old baby with persistent episodes of hypoglycaemia. The baby is irritable and has hypertonia. Glucose 1.8 mmol/L; insulin 12 mU/l; growth hormone 20 mU/L; cortisol 400 nmol/L; free fatty acids are normal.

○ 2. A 3–week-old boy presents with hypoglycaemia. He has cryptorchidism and is not fixing and following.

○ 3. A 3-day-old infant with a birth weight of 4.8 kg has had a hypoglycaemic event. On examination the baby was macrosomic, had hepatosplenomegaly and an umbilical hernia.

answers

1. Type 1 diabetes mellitus

Answers: A D

The incidence of type 1 diabetes mellitus in childhood (0–14 years) is variable from one country to another. The incidence is thought to be increasing in some countries, particularly in the under 5 years age group. The incidence in the UK is 13.5 in 100, 000, in China 0.6 in 100, 000, and is at its highest in Finland at 42.9 in 100, 000. There is a family history of type 1 diabetes mellitus in 10% of cases. If a sibling has type 1, the risk to the index case is 8%; if the father has type 1 the risk is 5–6%; and if the mother has type 1 the risk is 2–3%. If both parents have type 1 the risk increases to 30%. At least one type of autoimmune antibody is found in the vast majority of patients at diagnosis. Islet cell antibodies (ICA) are found in 65–80% of newly diagnosed type 1 diabetics, glutamic acid decarboxylase (GAD) antibodies are found in 65–80%. The diabetes most commonly found in children with cystic fibrosis is cystic fibrosis-related diabetes (CFRD) which is a distinct entity from either type 1 or type 2 diabetes, however type 1 diabetes can be found to occur alongside cystic fibrosis.

2. G protein abnormalities

Answers: C E

There are three intracellular messenger pathways in which hormones may act, namely cyclic adenosine monophosphate (cAMP), intracellular calcium, or tyrosine kinase. Hormone receptors linked to cAMP do not generate cAMP directly but act via a G protein receptor on the cell surface. The G protein may be inhibitory (for example, somatostatin) or stimulatory (all other hormones). McCune–Albright syndrome and pseudohypoparathyroidism are disorders of hormone–receptor interactions. Vitamin D-dependent rickets and nephrogenic diabetes insipidus are syndromes of receptor resistance. De Morsier syndrome (also known as septo-optic dysplasia) is a developmental anomaly of the midline structures of the brain.

3. Gonadotrophins

Answers: C D E

The gonadotrophins, luteinizing hormone (LH) and follicle-stimulating hormone (FSH), are glycoproteins released form the anterior pituitary gland. They are composed of an α- and a β-subunit. In the male, Leydig cells respond to LH, which stimulates the first step in testosterone production. In the female, LH binds to ovarian cells and stimulates steroidogenesis. FSH binds to Sertoli cells in the male and increases the mass of the seminiferous tubules and supports the development of sperm. In the female, FSH binds to the glomerulosa cells and stimulates the conversion of testosterone to oestrogen. Gonadotrophin-releasing hormone (GnRH) stimulates the synthesis and secretion of LH and FSH. Expression and secretion of FSH are also inhibited by inhibin, which has no effect on LH. In the neonate there are high levels of gonadotrophins but these decline progressively until nocturnal increases occur leading up to the onset of puberty.

4. Pituitary gland hormones

Answers: B C D E

The pituitary gland consists of anterior and posterior component. The anterior pituitary gland arises from an outgrowth of ectoderm from the buccal mucosa. It secretes growth hormone, adrenocorticotrophic hormone (ACTH), thyroid-stimulating hormone (TSH), luteinising hormone (LH) and follicle-stimulating hormone (FSH). The posterior pituitary gland is derived from the down-growth of neural tissue and secretes vasopressin and prolactin. Gonadotrophin-releasing hormone is secreted by the hypothalamus into the portal circulation.

5. Physiological progression of puberty

Answer: B

The first sign of onset of puberty in girls is breast development. In boys it is the enlargement of the testicles to 4 ml. Up to 75% of boys will develop some degree of gynaecomastia as the rise in oestrogen levels initially exceeds that of testosterone. The majority of gynaecomastia settles spontaneously within 2 years, but some may require surgery if it persists and causes psychological problems. Following menarche in girls there is a marked deceleration in height velocity but not complete cessation of growth. In boys FSH stimulates Sertoli cells to promote spermatogenesis, and LH (luteinising hormone) stimulates Leydig cells to produce testosterone. In girls FSH stimulates the granulosa and theca cells to produce oestradiol, and LH stimulates the stromal cells to produce androgens.

6. Septo-optic dysplasia

Answers: A B C D

Septo-optic dysplasia is a developmental anomaly of the midline structures of the brain. It is classically characterised by: absence of septum pellucidum; optic nerve hypoplasia; pituitary hypoplasia with variable hormone deficiencies (most commonly this is growth hormone deficiency). These may be isolated or progress to an evolving endocrinopathy.

answers

7. Delayed puberty

Answer: All false

Delayed puberty is more common in boys. In both sexes the most common aetiology is constitutional delay of puberty. Klinefelter syndrome (47XXY) is associated with gynaecomastia and small testes, secondary to seminiferous tubule dysgenesis. The majority will enter puberty spontaneously but may need testosterone supplementation to achieve full virilisation. As they progress through puberty the need for treatment may be indicated by a raised FSH and later LH. Kallmann syndrome is associated with hypogonadotrophic hypogonadism and anosmia. If ovarian failure is the cause of delayed puberty the FSH and LH will be high as the hypothalamic–pituitary– gonadal axis attempts to hyper-stimulate the failing ovaries. Delayed puberty in boys with constitutional delay can be managed by observation alone in those patients that are happy with this plan. Those that are keen for treatment can be offered oxandrolone (a synthetic androgen) or testosterone. When testosterone is given the best route of administration is via intramuscular injection once a month. Oral testosterone is partially broken down by the gastrointestinal tract, leading to variable dose absorption, and there is little experience in puberty induction using testosterone patches.

8. Growth hormone insufficiency

Answers: B D E

Growth hormone (GH) is secreted in a pulsatile pattern and provocation tests of secretion are potentially hazardous. The gold standard test is the insulin tolerance test which should only be performed in specialist centres because of the risk of severe hypoglycaemia. Other provocation tests include the use of glucagon, arginine and clonidine. The oral glucose tolerance test is used to diagnose acromegaly.

9. Licensed indications for growth hormone

Answers: A B C D

Growth hormone deficiency, Turner syndrome, chronic renal failure, and Prader–Willi syndrome are all licensed indications for treatment with growth hormone. These recommendations have been endorsed by the National Institute for Clinical Excellence (NICE). Most regimens involve daily injections of the hormone.

10. Hyperthyroidism

Answers: A C

Neonatal hyperthyroidism is rare. It is caused by the transplacental transfer of maternal TSH receptor antibodies. Only a minority of babies (1.5%) born to mothers with Graves disease will be affected. Symptoms commonly occur at 24–48 hours of age but may be delayed for up to 10 days if maternal antithyroid drugs cross the placenta. Those severely affected have up to 25% mortality from cardiac arrhythmias and cardiac failure. Children with Graves disease with few exceptions have some enlargement of the thyroid gland. Hyperthyroidism may cause polyuria and nocturia due to increased glomerular filtration rate. The onset in childhood is usually insidious and has often been present for some time prior to diagnosis. Many of these children experience behavioural problems and school difficulties. Approximately 50% of children treated medically will be in long-term remission by 4 years, with a continued remission rate of 25% every 2 years after this up until 6 years of treatment. Persistently high thyroid antibody titres indicate a high chance of recurrence once the treatment is stopped. Favourable factors for long-term remission using medical treatment alone include the requirement for a low dose of antithyroid medication, a small goitre, lack of eye signs, and a lower initial free thyroxine (T_4). Antithyroid medication should be tapered and gradually withdrawn. Those requiring definitive treatment can be treated with radioactive iodine or thyroid surgery. The former is becoming more commonly used in paediatrics particularly in the USA and its safety profile to date has been very good.

11. Growth

Answers: A B C D E

Factors influencing intra-uterine growth include nutrition, genetic, maternal smoking, placental function, intra-uterine infections, and endocrine factors. There are three principal phases of post-natal growth. In infancy, it is predominantly influenced by nutrition; in childhood, growth hormone and thyroxine; and at puberty the sex hormones and growth hormone. However nutrition and GH influence growth at all stages. A child's height may be compared to the general population using centile charts and considered in terms of his/her genetic potential by comparison with the mid-parental height.

12. Cushing's syndrome

Answer: E

Cushing's syndrome is not common in childhood. The majority of cases are secondary to iatrogenic steroids given orally, by inhalation, intranasally, topically or intravenously. Other aetiologies include ACTH-secreting pituitary tumours (Cushing's disease), adrenal adenoma/carcinoma, adrenal hyperplasia and ectopic ACTH. A characteristic feature in childhood Cushing's is growth arrest. Simple obesity is associated with normal or advanced growth. The diagnosis of Cushing's syndrome in children is often difficult; this is because of the pulsatile nature in which the relevant hormones are secreted – 24-hour urinary free cortisols may appear normal on the first two collections and then show gross elevation when repeated 1 month later. Investigations include at least two 24-hour urinary free cortisols, 8 AM and 12 AM (midnight) cortisol and ACTH to look for loss of normal diurnal variation, and dexamethasone suppression tests. Sometimes it is necessary to do a corticotrophin-releasing hormone (CRH) test coupled with inferior petrosal sinus sampling to determine the aetiology. Cushing's syndrome with a low ACTH and failure to suppress cortisol with high-dose dexamethasone is likely to be secondary to adrenal pathology. A high ACTH and some cortisol and ACTH suppression with high-dose dexamethasone may be due to a pituitary abnormality. A high ACTH that does not suppress with high-dose dexamethasone may be secondary to ectopic ACTH. However, often the aetiology is rarely so clear cut and often the secreting tumours are difficult to pick up even with high resolution MRI.

13. Achondroplasia

Answers: A B C E

Achondroplasia has an autosomal dominant inheritance with 50% new mutations. Clinical features include megalocephaly, short limbs, prominent forehead, thoracolumbar kyphosis and mid-facial hypoplasia. Complications include dental malocclusion, hydrocephalus and repeated otitis media.

14. Bone metabolism

Answer: E

The genes for PTH and calcitonin are both located on the short arm of chromosome 11. The primary function of PTH is to prevent hypocalcaemia. The immediate effect of an increase in PTH is increased calcium absorption and increased phosphate excretion in the kidney alongside osteoclastic bone resorption. The gastrointestinal effect is delayed by 1-2 days and occurs via increased synthesis of $1,25(OH)_2$ vitamin D. Vitamin D-dependent rickets is a rare cause of rickets. Type 1 is secondary to deficiency of 1α hydroxylation of 25 hydroxy vitamin D; type 2 is due to resistance of $1,25(OH)_2$ vitamin D. Both are treated with calcitriol, large doses are necessary in type 2. Vitamin D-deficient rickets is treated with vitamin D; hypophosphataemic rickets is treated with frequent doses of phosphate and also calcitriol as there is associated deficiency of 1α-hydroxylation of 25-hydroxyvitamin D. Bone disease of prematurity is thought to be predominantly caused by phosphate and/or calcium deficiency, and is treated with phosphate and calcium supplements. Peak bone mass is attained in the third decade of life. Positive influencing factors include exercise, obesity, calcium, calcitonin, oestrogen, growth hormone (GH) and Afro-Caribbean race. Negative influencing factors include inactivity, malabsorption, anorexia, tumour necrosis factor(TNF)α, interleukin 1, glucocorticoids, vitamin D, PTH and Chinese and Caucasian race.

15. Tall stature

Answers: B C E

Klinefelter syndrome is defined as a karyotype of 47XXY and is associated with cryptorchidism, gynaecomastia, mental retardation, azoospermia, and infertility.

A karyotype of 45XO/46XY is associated with short stature. Marfan syndrome has an autosomal dominant inheritance. The clinical features include arachnodactyly, tall stature, scoliosis, high-arched palate, and joint hypermobility. Other associations are learning difficulties, lens dislocation, aortic dissection and mitral valve prolapse, and pneumothorax. The androgen excess of untreated congenital adrenal hyperplasia (CAH) leads to tall stature in childhood.

16. Survival rates of childhood malignancies

Answers: A B

The growth hormone axis is the most vulnerable to damage by radiotherapy. The function of the rest of the anterior pituitary is relatively resistant. Deficiencies of ACTH, gonadotrophin, and thyroid stimulating hormone (TSH) may occur up to 10 years after treatment, requiring long-term vigilance and follow-up. Growth can be affected in numerous ways after oncological treatment: for example, as a direct effect of radiotherapy on the spine; by damage to the hypothalamic–pituitary axis with growth hormone deficiency; by gonadal damage resulting in impaired pubertal growth; and by direct damage to the growth plates from both chemotherapy and radiotherapy. The ovary appears to be more resistant than the testis to chemotherapy but both may be damaged by radiotherapy. Alkylating agents such as cyclophosphamide cause damage to the germinal epithelium, resulting in azoospermia and infertility. Testosterone production from the Leydig cells is not generally affected by chemotherapy but is affected by direct radiotherapy.

17. Obesity

Answer: B

Obesity in childhood may be associated with several syndromes, the most common of which include Laurence–Moon–Biedl syndrome, Down syndrome, Prader–Willi syndrome and pseudohypoparathyroidism.
Laurence–Moon–Biedl is associated with polydactyly and clinodactyly. A short fourth metacarpal may indicate pseudohypoparathyroidism. Leptin is a hormone that is secreted from adipose tissue. It plays a role in the feeling of satiety, mediating appetite suppression action via the hypothalamus. Levels of leptin positively correlate with body fat and they are increased in obese people. Disorders of leptin can be a primary cause of obesity but are very rare. Therapeutic trials using leptin in simple obesity have been disappointing. Simple obesity results in rapid growth and development and is associated with an advanced bone age. Children < 3 years with simple obesity and non-obese parents are at low risk of obesity in adulthood. Parental obesity more than doubles the risk of adult obesity in young children; as children get older, the presence of obesity becomes an ever-increasingly important predictor of adult obesity. Patients with a craniopharyngioma very frequently have a problem with weight gain post-operatively. It is thought that this is due to the role of the hypothalamus in disturbance of satiety.

18. Adrenal gland

Answers: B C D

The adrenals are triangular in shape and located at the superior pole of the kidneys. Each adrenal gland comprises a cortex arising from the mesoderm at the cranial end of the mesonephros and a medulla which arises from neural crest cells. The cortex consists of three zones: the zona glomerulosa produces aldosterone; the zona fasciculata produces cortisol and androstenedione; and the zona reticularis produces dehydroepiandrosterone sulphate (DHEAS). The secretion of aldosterone is primarily regulated by the renin–angiotensin system. However, adrenocorticotrophic hormone (ACTH) can produce a temporary rise in aldosterone, but this is not sustained.

19. Diabetes insipidus

Answers: D E

Familial pituitary diabetes insipidus (DI) is most commonly inherited in an autosomal dominant form due to a mutation in one allele of the gene that encodes for vasopressin–neurophysin 2. When managing a child with cranial DI a careful search must be undertaken to look for aetiology. Sometimes the underlying pathology may not be apparent at the outset. A cranial MRI must be included in the work-up and repeated at 6–12-month intervals to detect latent histiocytosis or dysgerminoma. Cranial DI should never be assumed to be idiopathic. A cortisol or thyroid deficiency can mask DI and it is important to remember this in children with potential pan-hypopituitarism. Treatment with glucocorticoids peri-operatively in a child with a craniopharyngioma may reveal DI, and fluid balance must be very carefully managed. Vasopressin is produced in the supraoptic and paraventricular nuclei of the hypothalamus; it is transported along the supraoptic hypophyseal tract and stored in the posterior pituitary. The classic triphasic craniopharyngioma post-operative response is initial DI caused by resection of the pituitary stalk, SIADH due to release of stored vasopressin, followed by persistent DI. Nephrogenic DI is X-linked (V2 receptor gene mutation) or autosomal recessive (aquaporin 2 gene mutation). Although it seems paradoxical it can be treated with thiazide diuretics, amiloride or prostaglandin synthetase inhibitor to decrease urine solute load and hence decrease urine output.

20. Delayed puberty

Answers: A E

Kallman syndrome is hypogonadotrophic hypogonadism with anosmia and hence leads to pubertal delay. 5-α-reductase deficiency is a cause of ambiguous genitalia as the enzyme is used to convert testosterone to dihydrotestosterone. Polycystic ovaries are associated with insulin resistance, obesity and hirsutism. McCune–Albright syndrome may cause gonadotrophin-independent precocious puberty by spontaneous ovarian activation.

21. Precocious/pseudoprecocious puberty

Answers: A B D E

McCune–Albright syndrome is associated with gonadotrophin-independent precocious puberty in which the sex steroids are secreted by the gonads without gonadotrophin stimulation. Other characteristic features of the syndrome include irregular patches of skin pigmentation and polyostotic fibrous dysplasia of the bones. Simple virilising congenital adrenal hyperplasia (CAH) can present in both boys and girls in mid-childhood with signs of virilisation. It is important to exclude when diagnosing exaggerated physiological adrenarche. Centrally mediated precocious puberty (CPP) is more common in girls; in girls over the age of 6 years; it is often idiopathic. In the younger age group it is more likely to have a sinister aetiology, such as adrenal, ovarian or cranial tumours. In boys idiopathic CPP is rare and it is necessary to look hard for a causative factor; cranial imaging in this group is mandatory. CPP can be suppressed by GnRH agonists. When given in pharmacological doses they down-regulate GnRH receptors and consequently inhibit LH and FSH secretion. CPP is more common in children born prematurely who have had an intracranial haemorrhage, in children who have had cranial neoplasms, cranial irradiation, or raised intracranial pressure. This is due to premature activation (or premature release of inhibition) of GnRH release.

22. Turner syndrome

Answers: A B E

Turner syndrome is defined as having a 45XO karyotype and is associated with short stature, ovarian dysgenesis, and dysmorphic features. The clinical features include neonatal lymphoedema, short stature (mean adult height is 142 cm), widely spaced nipples, shield-shaped chest, ptosis, low posterior hair-line, webbed neck, wide carrying angle, and hyper-convex nails. There is a risk of developing autoimmune diseases (hypothyroidism, type 2 diabetes) and an association with horseshoe kidneys, coarctation of the aorta, and excessive pigmented naevi.

23. B: Chromosomes

Turner syndrome is due to complete or partial absence of one of the X chromosomes in a female. It must always be excluded in any female presenting with short stature. The incidence is 1 in 2500 live-born girls. There may not be any apparent dysmorphic features and it has been diagnosed late in adult women presenting to gynaecological clinics with difficulty conceiving. The possible dysmorphic features include: pedal oedema, low hair-line, neck webbing, high-arched palate, widely spaced nipples leading to a shield-shaped chest, café-au-lait spots, cubitus valgus, hyper-convex nails, short fourth and fifth metacarpals, associated cardiac defects (eg coarctation) and renal anomalies (eg horseshoe kidney). Up to 20% of girls may spontaneously enter puberty and may achieve menses, but the majority require oestrogen therapy. Those that have spontaneous puberty should be warned that it does not mean they will produce ova. There are now many women with Turner syndrome who have had a pregnancy following in-vitro fertilisation (IVF) with a donor egg. In view of this it is essential to introduce oestrogen therapy gradually, to ensure adequate breast and uterine development. These girls need to be followed up and investigated for possible thyroid problems, middle-ear disease, hypertension and insulin resistance. Learning difficulties may occur, particularly in the areas of maths and geography. Hypothyroidism does result in short stature but usually children are overweight if they have this. Coeliac disease in young children often presents with symptoms but can be asymptomatic with poor growth as a manifestation; such children will often have a weight centile lower than their height centile. Full blood count and C reactive protein may be abnormal, but are unlikely in this case to lead to a specific diagnosis.

24. B: Septo-optic dysplasia

The hypoglycaemia could have been caused by any of the diagnoses listed. However, with both glycogen storage disease and galactosaemia other clinical signs would have been expected, such as hepatomegaly, and in galactosaemia failure to thrive and cataracts. A diagnosis of hyper-insulinaemic hypoglycaemia would cause a high birth weight which was not present in this child. The problems with fixing and following could not be explained by MCAD but could be explained by a diagnosis of septo-optic dysplasia, which is a developmental anomaly of the mid-line structures of the brain. It is classically characterised by absence of the septum pellucidum, optic nerve hypoplasia, and pituitary hypoplasia with variable pituitary hormone deficiencies. Deficiency of either GH or ACTH can lead to hypoglycaemia.

25. C: Hypothyroidism

Acquired hypothyroidism usually has an insidious onset. There is associated increase in weight gain and reduced height velocity. Lack of energy, cold intolerance, constipation, and dry skin and hair are often presenting features. Most children will change shoe size once or twice a year if they have a normal growth velocity; often parents are more aware of shoe size change than change in height. High levels of thyroid-stimulating hormone (TSH) may cross react with follicle-stimulating hormone (FSH) receptors, leading to breast development. School performance usually remains normal. Addison's disease is associated with poor weight gain and hypotension. Cushing syndrome is associated with androgenisation secondary to over-stimulation of the adrenal glands, hypertension and plethoric facies. Chronic fatigue syndrome commonly results in poor school attendance and is not associated with decreased growth but may be associated with increased weight gain secondary to inactivity. Constitutional delay of growth and puberty may result in poor weight and height gain. Girls that are overweight tend to enter puberty early rather than late, and have associated pubic hair following initial breast development.

26. D: Klinefelter syndrome

Constitutional tall stature occurs in a child with tall parents and is associated with a centile position appropriate for the mid-parental predicated centile. Marfan syndrome is not associated with cryptorchidism but is associated with tall stature relative to the mid-parental predicted centile. Soto syndrome is an overgrowth syndrome with excessive linear growth in the first few years of life, which then characteristically falls back. McCune–Albright syndrome can be associated with tall stature due to thyrotoxicosis, excess of GH, or precocious puberty, but could not explain the appearance of the genitalia. Klinefelter syndrome is associated with tall stature, gynaecomastia and cryptorchidism.

27. B: Ultrasound scan of the pelvis

An ultrasound scan of the pelvis will give the most immediate information as to what the diagnosis might be. It will be possible to tell if there are internal female genitalia, and you can also look for undescended testes. 17-OHP is very important and needs to be done to rule out congenital adrenal hyperplasia (CAH). All babies have a surge of 17-OHP following delivery and the level is best done 4 days after birth to avoid falsely high results; however, in this situation it should be done on the same day – but be aware of false positives. Most laboratories will be unable to give a result on the day that the sample is taken. U&E will be normal at day 2 even if the diagnosis is CAH. Babies who present with a collapse secondary to CAH usually present on about day 10 with a salt-losing crisis. Karyotype is an important investigation in this baby but you will not get an answer the same day. It is important to explain to the parents that the chromosomal sex is not the most important determining factor in deciding the sex of rearing.

28. BASIC SCIENCE OF HORMONES

1.   **B – Thyroid hormone**
2.   **G – Luteinising hormone**
3.   **H – Aldosterone**

Hormones are chemical messengers produced by a variety of specialized cells. There are three main types of hormones, namely, amine, steroid, and peptide. Hormones may be secreted in a continuous (eg thyroxine) or an intermittent pattern (FSH , LH, GH, prolactin, cortisol, ACTH). The hormones secreted by the anterior pituitary gland are luteinising hormone (LH), follicle-stimulating hormone (FSH), growth hormone, adrenocorticotrophic hormone (ACTH) and thyroid-stimulating hormone (TSH). In the male, LH binds to Leydig cells and stimulates the first step in testosterone production. In the female it binds to ovarian cells and stimulates steroidogenesis. FSH binds to the Sertoli cells in the male and increases the mass of the seminiferous tubules and supports the development of sperm. In the female, FSH binds to the glomerulosa cells and stimulates the conversion of testosterone to oestrogen. Growth hormone has a pulsatile secretion pattern consisting of peaks and troughs and acts via the second messenger of insulin-like growth factor(IGF)-1. TSH is a trophic hormone and causes the release and production of thyroid hormone, T_4. ACTH is responsible for stimulation of the adrenal cortex and in particular the production of cortisol. It produces a temporary rise in aldosterone but this is not sustained. Aldosterone is primarily regulated by the renin–angiotensin system, in response to electrolyte balance and plasma volumes. The adrenal cortex has three principal functions: glucocorticoid production (cortisol) in the zona fasciculata; mineralocorticoid production (aldosterone) in the zona glomerulosa; androgen production (testosterone, DHEAS) in the zona reticularis.

29. PITUITARY HORMONE TESTING

1.   J – Hypothalamic dysfunction

The presence of a craniopharyngioma and its surgical excision may lead to hypothalamic damage. Hypothalamic disorders are characterised by effects on the appetite leading to hyperphagia and also problems with temperature and thirst control.

2.   D – Combined hypothalamic and pituitary hormone abnormalities

The insulin tolerance test causes a fall in the blood glucose, which in turn stimulates the release of counter-regulatory hormones if the glucose concentration falls below 2.6 mmol/L. Two of the counter-regulatory hormones are growth hormone (GH) and cortisol. The GH is released from the pituitary gland and the cortisol is released by the adrenal glands under the control of pituitary-released adrenocorticotrophic hormone (ACTH). The table shows that despite the low blood glucose concentration there is no significant change in GH or cortisol release, which—in light of the clinical history—is suggestive of pituitary dysfunction. The baseline concentration of thyroid stimulating hormone (TSH) is within the normal range; however, although there is an initial rise following the thyrotrophin-releasing hormone under normal thyroid regulation, the concentration should have fallen by a time of 60 minutes. Its continued rise implies damage to this regulation and in view of the normal baseline TSH concentration is suggestive of this problem being at a hypothalamic level.

3.   F – Gonadotrophin deficiency

Kallman syndrome is hypogonadotrophic hypogonadism associated with anosmia.

30. HYPOGLYCAEMIA

1. A – Hyper-insulinaemic hypoglycaemia

The baby has hyperinsulinaemic hypoglycaemia as the insulin concentration should be zero in the presence of hypoglycaemia (i.e. glucose < 2.6 mmol/L). This is occurring at 6 weeks of age and hence is of too long a duration to be a transient hyperinsulinaemia as seen in the infant of a diabetic mother.

2. D – Galactosaemia

Glycogen storage diseases and enzyme deficiencies like galactosaemia cause hypoglycaemia due to inadequate glucose production and may be associated with other system involvement. The inability to fix and follow would be consistent with cataracts.

3. I – Beckwith–Wiedemann syndrome

A macrosomic baby is associated with hyperinsulinism, which may be persistent or transient. Beckwith–Wiedemann syndrome is a cause of transient neonatal hyperinsulinism and is also associated with macrosomia and umbilical hernia.

Evidence-based medicine, clinical governance, surgery and consent

Robert Wheeler

Multiple Choice Questions

1. An irreducible inguinal hernia in a boy infant

○ A should be treated with gallows traction
○ B requires herniotomy within 6 hours
○ C can be expected to resolve with sedation
○ D will reduce spontaneously under general anaesthesia
○ E is a direct cause of testicular damage

2. Meckel's diverticulum

○ A is distinguishable from a gut duplication on radioisotope scanning
○ B is implicated in gut obstruction
○ C is sited in the jejunum
○ D causes bleeding by generating excessive acid in the stomach
○ E presents with an umbilical discharge

3. Intussusception

○ A characteristically presents in the 5–10-year-old age group
○ B presents in a similar way to rectal prolapse
○ C will, in the majority of cases, recur
○ D requires antibiotic administration
○ E will usually not respond to pneumatic reduction

4. Pyloric stenosis

○ A is more common in boys
○ B presents with a hyperchloraemic alkalosis
○ C presents with green vomitus
○ D Is associated with coffee-ground vomitus
○ E causes aciduria

5. Inguinal hernias in boy infants aged less than 1 year

- ○ A can be managed with a truss
- ○ B will resolve spontaneously in 10–20% of cases
- ○ C are usually bilateral
- ○ D recur after herniotomy
- ○ E require analysis of the sex chromosomes

6. Acute appendicitis

- ○ A is a fatal disease
- ○ B is associated with urinary symptoms
- ○ C may be treated with antibiotics alone for a period of weeks
- ○ D is associated with a fulminant illness in infants aged over 1 year
- ○ E is a clinical diagnosis

7. Hypospadias

- ○ A describes an imperfect location of the urethral meatus in boys or girls
- ○ B is associated with inter-sex states
- ○ C is associated with abnormalities of the ureter or kidney
- ○ D is a heritable condition
- ○ E is associated with difficulties in coitus

8. Umbilical hernias in children aged under 5 years

- ○ A usually resolve spontaneously
- ○ B are not, typically, painful or tender
- ○ C are less likely to resolve spontaneously in the Afro-Caribbean than in the Caucasian population
- ○ D become irreducible
- ○ E share clinical features with supra-umbilical hernias

9. External angular dermoid cysts

- ○ A characteristically resolve spontaneously
- ○ B are located at the inner canthus of the eye
- ○ C erode the underlying skull table
- ○ D represent mesodermal inclusion tissue
- ○ E are congenital

10. Green vomitus in infants

- ○ A is not precisely synonymous with bilious vomiting associated with gut obstruction
- ○ B is considered a sinister sign
- ○ C is suggestive of pyloric stenosis
- ○ D is characteristic of gut obstruction
- ○ E is pathognomonic of midgut volvulus

11. Caldicott Guardians

○ A represent a trust's corporate responsibility for data protection
○ B are appointed by the local authority
○ C acquire parental responsibility on behalf of a trust
○ D were created as a result of the Children Act 1989
○ E are only responsible for the electronically stored parts of a child's hospital record

12. Parental responsibility

○ A is automatically acquired by the woman who gives birth to a baby
○ B is transferred to the local authority as a result of a care order
○ C is lost by the birth mother if her baby is adopted
○ D is lost by the mother when the child reaches majority (18 years of age in the UK)
○ E is lost by the mother when the child becomes Gillick competent

13. The capacity for a child to consent for treatment

○ A is recognised by Act of Parliament in a 16-year-old
○ B requires court approval before 16 years
○ C is considered with equal weight for assent or refusal at 15 years
○ D was challenged by Gillick & Sons (Solicitors) in 1983
○ E is not accepted below the age of 12 years

14. Anorectal malformations in neonates

○ A are not associated with abnormalities of the urinary system
○ B are associated with pre-sacral masses
○ C do not need to be excluded in cases of oesophageal atresia
○ D are associated with urinary incontinence
○ E make imaging of the lumbosacral spine mandatory

15. Sacrococcygeal teratomas

○ A are congenital
○ B usually have benign histology at birth
○ C are associated with fetal death
○ D are invariably associated with a high α-fetoprotein in the first week of life
○ E are located at any point along the vertebral column

16. Pectus excavatum

○ A is characterised by dyspnoea at rest
○ B is associated with chest pain
○ C is associated with congenital diaphragmatic hernia
○ D resolves spontaneously
○ E responds to physiotherapy

17. Midgut malrotation

- ○ A Is synonymous with midgut volvulus
- ○ B is associated with gastroschisis
- ○ C is a clinical diagnosis
- ○ D responds to prolonged therapy with pro-kinetic agents
- ○ E is not diagnosed by the use of ultrasound

18. Tracheo-oesophageal fistula (TOF)

- ○ A usually presents during the second year of life
- ○ B is more common in Scandinavia than in the UK
- ○ C follows a Mendelian pattern of inheritance
- ○ D is not associated with gastro-oesophageal reflux
- ○ E is usually detected antenatally

19. Preputial phimosis

- ○ A will usually resolve spontaneously by puberty
- ○ B is not caused by lichen sclerosis et atrophicus
- ○ C responds permanently to topical steroids
- ○ D is common in both sexes
- ○ E is physiological

20. Foster parents

- ○ A share parental responsibility with the local authority
- ○ B can only provide for short-term fostering arrangements
- ○ C may be sourced from the private sector (as opposed to the local authority)
- ○ D have the right to refuse to return the child to its natural parents
- ○ E are paid for their services

Best of Five Questions

21. An 18-month-old boy presents with vomiting, abdominal pain and rectal bleeding. He is dehydrated and there is an abdominal mass. A Meckel's scan is negative. What is the MOST likely diagnosis?

- A Enteric duplication
- B Intussusception
- C Meckel's diverticulum
- D Midgut volvulus
- E Appendicitis

22. An 8-year-old boy presents with abdominal pain and bile-stained vomit. A contrast study of the upper gastrointestinal tract reveals his duodenojejunal flexure is lying in the midline. No mass is palpable in the abdomen. Which is the MOST likely diagnosis?

- A Intussusception
- B Appendicitis
- C Colonic carcinoma
- D Midgut malrotation
- E Adhesion obstruction

23. A 6-year-old boy has a healthy prepuce, which is 60% adherent to the glanular surface. What is the BEST treatment?

- A Divide the adhesions in outpatients
- B Divide the adhesions under general anaesthesia
- C Circumcise
- D Allow for spontaneous resolution
- E Use steroid creams

24. Legal consent for the ritual circumcision of a 10-year-old boy is BEST obtained in which way?

- A From the biological mother
- B From both parents
- C Over the telephone
- D From the boy if he is Gillick competent
- E Orally, rather than in writing

25. Inguinal hernias in premature boy infants are MOST likely to

- A Resolve spontaneously
- B Result in testicular atrophy
- C Recur after surgery
- D Transform into hydrocoeles
- E Be direct hernias

answers

1. Inguinal hernia in boys

Answers: D E

Irreducible inguinal hernias may exert pressure on the spermatic cord and compromise testicular blood supply, resulting in testicular ischaemia. Herniotomy, the operation to cure the hernia, is ideally performed several days after the hernia is reduced. This delay allows local inguinal oedema to resolve and reduces the chances of operative injury to the cord. Gallows traction, relying on gravity to reduce the hernia, is no longer used. The hernia should be reduced immediately on arrival at hospital using firm but gentle pressure to squeeze the sac contents back into the abdomen. This closed procedure may take 10–15 minutes and can be very difficult, often requiring sedation and supervision by a senior. Only babies in whom closed reduction has failed should have open surgery as an emergency. Even in this group, many irreducible hernias reduce spontaneously during induction of anaesthesia.

2. Meckel's diverticulum

Answer: B

Meckel's diverticulum is sited in the distal ileum, and is lined by ectopic gastric mucosa. The mucosa produces acid which may ulcerate the adjacent diverticular and ileal mucosa, causing enteric bleeding or perforation. The ectopic gastric mucosa takes up and excretes technetium-99 pertechnetate, so can be detected by scintigraphy. However, false-positive results occur because this isotope also images duplication cysts, gastrogenic cysts and Barrett's oesophagus. The diverticulum may be connected to the umbilicus by a band of fibrous tissue, which may cause gut obstruction. This band is the remnant of the omphalomesenteric duct. If the duct is patent, then a connection between the gut and the skin is formed, allowing umbilical leakage. However, in these circumstances the diverticulum is no longer blindly ended, and would therefore be defined as a fistula.

3. Intussusception

Answers: B D

Intussusception is characteristically a disease of infants up to 1 year, although it is described in older children. It usually presents with screaming, pain, rectal bleeding and an abdominal mass. However, the apex of the intussusception may occasionally protrude through the anus. About 5–10% will recur whether treated by pneumatic reduction or by open surgery. Intussusception is a serious disease that is fatal if inadequately treated. Full resuscitation with fluids and antibiotics is mandatory before any attempt at either closed or operative reduction is made. Closed reduction using a pneumatic technique under radiological control should have a success rate in the order of 90%.

4. Pyloric stenosis

Answers: A D E

Infantile hypertrophic pyloric stenosis (IHPS) is four times as common in boys as it is in girls. As the pyloric narrowing is proximal to the biliary outflow tract, bile-stained vomit is not seen. Bile stained vomiting should be considered as mutually exclusive with the diagnosis of IHPS. The persistent vomiting of IHPS causes loss of sodium, chloride, acid, water and potassium. Since sodium homeostasis takes precedence over that of hydrogen, in exchange for sodium the kidney excretes hydrogen ions. Paradoxical aciduria, in an alkalotic hypochloraemic patient, is thus observed. There is an associated gastritis that causes bleeding, hence brownish discoloration of the vomit (or even coffee-grounds vomit).

5. Inguinal hernia in boys

Answer: D

In infants aged up to 1 year hernias are unsuitable for non-operative management and only very rarely resolve spontaneously. They are usually unilateral in boys, but bilateral in up to 50% of girls. A contralateral metachronous hernia may develop in up to 20% of patients. Hernias can recur after surgery, notably in premature infants (5%), and in children with connective tissue disease. Due to the association with androgen insensitivity, phenotypically female infants with inguinal hernias must undergo karyotype analysis.

6. Acute appendicitis

Answer: All true

Appendicitis still causes death in children, usually because of late diagnosis. The inflamed appendix may be adherent to or adjacent to the urinary bladder, which may give symptoms of urinary frequency. Bacterial translocation may occur across the adherent viscous walls and result in bacteruria and pyuria. This is one of many situations that can lead to a delay in diagnosis. If the appendicitis is untreated, necrosis of the appendix wall leads to perforation. In infants over 1 year, the omental mechanism for walling off the perforation and inflammatory process may be inadequate. Generalised peritonitis and a potentially fulminant illness can result. In the older child, provided the perforation and inflammation remain localised, an appendix mass forms. This mass tends to arise out of the pelvis, and is hazardous to operate on. A

answers

prolonged course of antibiotics, guided by blood cultures, is administered (initially intravenously and subsequently orally). With this treatment the perforation usually heals spontaneously after 6–8 weeks. Once the infection and inflammation have resolved, interval appendectomy is performed. Laboratory tests are not specific for diagnosing appendicitis. Ultrasound may describe an image that is consistent with acute appendicitis, but the main role of ultrasound scanning is to demonstrate an associated abscess.

7. Hypospadias

Answers: A B D E

Hypospadias in boys involves a ventral urinary meatus, but this is almost always associated with a hooded dorsal foreskin that is deficient ventrally. Additionally, the ventral skin is often tight, leading to a bent erection. In girls, hypospadias means the recession of the urethral meatus proximally up the anterior wall of the vagina. Penile hypospadias is one of the major features of the genetic ambiguity encountered in inter-sex states. Male hypospadias often runs in families, although Mendelian inheritance is only one of a variety of proposed aetiologies. Others include the ingestion of anti-androgenic medications (such as cimetidine) during pregnancy, and the ingestion of increasing amounts of oestrogens. Coitus may be difficult with a substantially bent erection. Hypospadias is not associated with upper tract pathology.

8. Umbilical hernias

Answers: A B D E

Umbilical hernias usually resolve spontaneously, given time. The herniation occurs through a circular scar, and scars almost always contract, hence the hole will close. The process of closure may continue up to puberty, but if the child is teased about it, or the parents put pressure on the surgeon, surgical closure is performed. Surgical preferences vary widely, but there is some consensus for repairing the hernia when the child is 4–7 years old, if requested. The hernia may cause symptoms of discomfort, but rarely becomes irreducible. Both umbilical and supra-umbilical hernias present with a bulge in the umbilical region. The umbilical hernia tends to bulge outwards, through a circular defect in the abdominal wall. The supra-umbilical variety emerges from a linear defect and bulges downwards.

9. External angular dermoid cysts

Answers: C E

External angular dermoids result from ectodermal tissue that is trapped and buried between the advancing plates of facial mesoderm, which fuse at the lateral margin of the orbit. They continue to grow inexorably, and may erode the tables of the skull, to lie on the dura of the anterior cranial fossa. There is no tendency to resolve, although they do occasionally rupture. The spillage of the contents causes a local inflammatory reaction, but the cyst reforms and continues to grow, as the ectodermal lining continues to produce secretions.

10. Green vomitus

Answers: B D

As it emerges from the ampulla, bile has a fluorescent yellow colour. If it cannot flow distally because of high gut obstruction bile will reflux into the stomach. Contact with the gastric secretions turns it into a green colour. Infants who vomit green fluid have gut obstruction until proved otherwise. Because of this, bilious vomiting in infants is a marker of sinister pathology. The principal causes of gut obstruction in this age group, such as volvulus, intussusception, incarcerated hernia (and atresia, meconium ileus and Hirschsprung disease in neonates) are all very poorly tolerated. Because of relatively fragile homeostasis in this age group, these can all be devastating illnesses. For this reason, paediatricians are encouraged to fear bile-stained vomit and to refer early.

11. Caldicott Guardians

Answer: A

The Caldicott Guardians were appointed by health authorities and trusts following the publication of a report of the 'Review of Patient-Identifiable Information' by Caldicott in 1997 (for the Department of Health). Guardians are usually senior clinicians and their responsibility is to safeguard confidentiality. According to the Data Protection Act 1998, all written and electronic patient information is included within their responsibility. Guardians may also have a duty to maintain the general obligation of confidentiality shared by all healthcare workers within the trust. There is no relationship with paediatric practice beyond the obvious responsibility of ensuring that the principles of data protection are followed when handling paediatric patient data.

12. Parental responsibility

Answers: A C D

Parental responsibility is automatically conferred on the woman who gives birth to the baby. The child's father acquires parental responsibility provided that he is married to the mother, and his parental responsibility dates from that marriage. For babies born after 1/12/2003, an unmarried father also acquires parental responsibility if his name is registered on the birth certificate. Parental responsibility can only be transferred away from a parent by adoption. It may be shared with a local authority, but it is not transferable. The mother retains her rights and responsibilities during the period when the child is subject to a care order. Parental responsibility survives until the child reaches majority, although priority is often given to the views of a competent adolescent. A child's capacity for decision-making may therefore have a bearing on the extent to which that child is permitted to exercise autonomy, but this does not negate parental responsibility.

13. Capacity for consent

Answer: A

The Family Law Reform Act 1969 conferred the right to consent to treatment on 16- and 17-year-olds, although they have not yet reached the age of majority (18 years in the UK). Children can provide valid consent at any age if they can be shown to be competent to make the particular decision with which they are faced. Their competence ('capacity') is assessed according to the criteria established during the Victoria Gillick case. The child must therefore be able to understand the nature and need for the procedure, the risks and benefits, the consequences of not having the procedure, and the alternatives available. All these issues need to be discussed in language that the child can understand. The assessor, who will be the senior doctor taking consent, must be satisfied that the child can retain these concepts for long enough to consider them carefully, so being able to come to a firm conclusion. If the child is found to be 'Gillick competent' then no further consent from parents is required. However, it is vital that the seriousness of the proposed treatment is taken into consideration. While 8-year-olds might have capacity to consent for a venepuncture, it is less likely that they are competent to agree to repair of an inguinal hernia. Similarly, 13-year-olds may demonstrate capacity to consent to an emergency appendectomy, but might struggle to demonstrate capacity to consent for a course of cytotoxic chemotherapy. In general terms, the Gillick doctrine is applied to assent rather than dissent. Parental responsibility is retained until the child reaches the age of 18 years, and during all of this time a parent can supply the consent that is required for treatment, even against the wishes of a Gillick-competent dissenter. Just how strongly the treatment is enforced depends on the seriousness of the illness. A child in this category may well be permitted to 'escape' treatment for a scarred foreskin if they are sufficiently determined. However, the courts will not permit a child to die of treatable disease merely because they refuse to cooperate.

14. Anorectal malformations

Answers: B D E

Urinary tract anomalies occur in more than 40% of all patients with anorectal malformations. Amongst other urinary complications, 10% of those with low anorectal anomalies and 30% of those with high anomalies will suffer from urinary incontinence. Children with the most extreme forms of malformation (eg cloaca or rectovesical fistula) can be expected to have a 90% chance of an associated genitourinary abnormality. Sacral deformities and lumbar vertebral anomalies are also common. Their identification prompts closer consideration of the possibility of a neurogenic bladder or bowel. Currarino syndrome/triad describes the association of anorectal anomalies, sacral anomalies and pre-sacral masses, such as anterior meningocoeles, teratomas or enteric duplications. Anorectal anomalies are grouped with vertebral, tracheo-oesophageal, renal and radial anomalies, within the VATER complex. The presentation of any one of these anomalies should prompt a search for the other features.

15. Sacrococcygeal teratomas

Answers: A B C D

Sacrococcygeal teratomas are located only in the sacrococcygeal region. In 10% there may be only a pre-sacral component, with no external sign of their presence. Derived from germ cells, teratomas are often located in the midline. This is due to a failure of some of these pluripotential cells to successfully migrate from the extra-embryonic yolk sac to their target organs, the gonads. The result is tumour formation within the brain, mediastinum, retroperitoneum, and sacrococcygeal regions. Germ cells that successfully migrate can still develop abnormally, forming teratomas (among other tumours) within the testis or ovary. Sacrococcygeal teratomas are the most common germ cell tumours in children, and are three times more common in girls. Some 80% are benign. The younger the age of post-natal diagnosis, the more likely the tumour is to be benign. A large sacrococcygeal teratoma may cause high-output cardiac failure in the fetus, as a result of tumour vascular steal. The resulting hydrops may result in fetal death, and has prompted attempts to perform in-utero resections. It is thought that 50% of fetuses with this condition die by week 20 of gestation. Levels of α-fetoprotein are invariably high in all newborn babies, whether or not they have a teratoma.

16. Pectus excavatum

Answers: B C D

Pectus excavatum is strongly associated with connective tissues disorders, and with syndromes in which these disorders occur, such as Marfan syndrome. It is also seen often in survivors of repaired congenital diaphragmatic hernia. About 30–40% of patients with pectus complain of chest wall pain and tenderness. Pectus excavatum can resolve, although this is rare and may be because many patients simply become resigned to the presence of their deformity. For those in whom the condition does not resolve, surgery may be an option. There is little evidence that pectus deformities have any effect on cardiorespiratory function. The indications for surgery are therefore limited to the cosmetic and social problems associated with thoracic deformity. Minimally invasive pectus surgery is more likely to be considered by many adolescents who might have been discouraged by the invasiveness of the previously available open repair technique.

17. Midgut malrotation

Answer: B

Midgut malrotation describes the situation where the bowel is abnormally and incompletely fixed to the posterior abdominal wall. It may be due to an interruption of the dual process of gut rotation and fixation that should occur as the bowel re-enters the abdominal cavity during the first trimester of pregnancy. The consequence of the anomaly is that the bowel, incompletely fixed to the posterior abdominal wall, is abnormally mobile. This mobility means that there is a tendency for the midgut to twist around the mesenteric vessels. These act as a pivot for the twist, because they are connected to the great vessels that are firmly fixed to the posterior abdominal wall. The twisting process, described as volvulus, occludes the mesenteric vessels and may cause midgut infarction unless rapidly treated. An abdominal wall defect, such as gastroschisis and exomphalos, would be expected to interfere with the process of gut fixation. The incidence of midgut malrotation in these patients is very high, so it is regarded as an intrinsic part of those abnormalities. The diagnosis is made radiologically. Ultrasound may reveal an abnormal anatomical relationship between the superior mesenteric artery and vein, suggesting malrotation. However, contrast studies of the upper gastrointestinal (the duodenal loop and the duodenojejunal flexure) remain the gold standard for diagnosis. If doubt remains, laparotomy is required to confirm or refute the diagnosis, and perform corrective surgery if required. Medical therapy has no place in the treatment of malrotation, although thorough resuscitation is clearly vital in the management of volvulus.

18. Tracheo-oesophageal fistula

Answer: All false

Tracheo-oesophageal fistula (TOF) – and oesophageal atresia (OA) – usually present early in the neonatal period because the atresia component of the complex prevents swallowing. In at least 96% of cases oesophageal atresia accompanies the tracheo-oesophageal fistula. The rare isolated fistula can present outside infancy, usually as recurrent chest infection. There is no reported regional variation in this anomaly, nor is there evidence for a Mendelian pattern of inheritance. However, there are a number of reports of multiple family members with the diagnosis. Gastro-oesophageal reflux (GER) has been demonstrated in 50% of patients within 5 years of repair of their TOF/OA. Symptoms of GER continue in 50% of adult survivors. A small stomach and polyhydramnios may be seen on antenatal ultrasound that may be indicative of OA. However, no antenatal marker exists for TOF.

19. Preputial phimosis

Answers: A E

Phimosis is derived from the Greek word to 'muzzle'. In this context it usually refers to a male foreskin that is insufficiently dilated to allow the glans penis to emerge through the preputial ring. When the phimosis resolves, the preputial ring has reached sufficient diameter to allow the prepuce to retract back across the glans and reach the coronal sulcus. In theory, phimosis applies to girls; the labia minora are the embryological equivalent to the preputial ring. Fusion of the labia minora is thus the female equivalent of the condition, although relatively few children are referred with this transient complaint. In both sexes, topical oestrogen application results in separation of the structures, but it recurs as soon as therapy is stopped. Phimosis is usually physiological and resolves by puberty. Circumcision of these children is therefore only very rarely appropriate. The phimosis may be caused by pathology, which usually manifests as scarring. The formation of cicatrix causes a tight and sometimes highly symptomatic phimosis, and is usually indicative of balanitis xerotica obliterans (BXO). This condition is closely allied histologically to lichen sclerosis et atrophicus. Recurrent infection, in the absence of BXO, is another cause of scarring. Both conditions necessitate circumcision.

20. Foster parents

Answers: C D E

Fostering may either be provided by private arrangement or by local authority foster parents. Both may provide either short-term or long-term fostering. Parental responsibility may be shared between the biological mother (and her husband if they are married) and the local authority. However, no element of parental responsibility is transferred to the foster parents. Strictly speaking, foster parents are empowered to refuse to hand over a child to a drunken parent who turns up on the doorstep in the middle of the night. However, in situations where the welfare of the child is at no immediate risk, foster parents have no right to retain the child against a parent's wishes. Foster parents are paid either by private arrangement or by the local authority. The weekly rate for fostering a child aged 11–15 years outside London in 1997 was £90.08.

21. B: Intussusception

In this age group intussusception is the leading diagnosis. A duplication cyst could give all these features, although it may contain sufficient gastric epithelium to produce a positive Meckel's scan. However, it would be a comparatively rare diagnosis. A Meckel's diverticulum is still possible (scintigraphy has poor sensitivity) and it could have bled, but there are also features of gut obstruction. Although Meckel's diverticulum can be the cause of gut obstruction, it is less likely to be bleeding and obstructing at the same time. Midgut volvulus is plausible and is important to consider in these circumstances. However, in this age group, it is less likely than intussusception. Acute appendicitis can certainly cause gut obstruction and a palpable mass, but rarely presents with rectal bleeding.

22. D: Midgut malrotation

This boy has gut obstruction. The abnormal siting of his duodenojejunal flexure (which should overlie or lie to the left of his left vertebral pedicles) indicates that by definition he has midgut malrotation. This can lead to gut obstruction by either the predisposition to midgut volvulus, or due to the abnormal peritoneal bands that are inherent to malrotation and can obstruct the bowel, whether or not there is an associated volvulus. The lack of an abdominal mass makes the first three diagnoses less likely, although it does not exclude them. Acute appendicitis would be the most likely diagnosis if not for the results of the contrast study. It is certainly possible that a child with uncomplicated malrotation could get appendicitis. Intussusception is unlikely in an 8-year-old, and carcinoma (although it has been recorded) is very rare. Adhesion obstruction is a common cause of gut obstruction, although absence of a past history of abdominal surgery reduces the likelihood.

23. D: Allow for spontaneous resolution

Preputial adhesions resolve. All of the above solutions are still in use in the UK in 2003. It is well recognised that if preputial adhesions are separated either by physical or chemical means, the vast majority subsequently re-form. Smegma may accumulate under the adherent prepuce, forming a 'preputial pearl'. Once the adhesion resolves, this mass of secretions is extruded with the urine. No pathology flows from the presence of preputial adhesions in children. This means that any invasive treatment is undesirable, and the level of undesirability is directly proportional to the invasiveness of the treatment. Whether division without anaesthesia is more or less invasive than that using general anaesthesia is a matter for debate.

24. B: From both parents

One consent is all that is required to protect a doctor from claims in negligence or from accusations of criminal common assault. The biological mother would be the most likely person to have parental responsibility for this child. Oral consent is perfectly adequate in law, but has the disadvantage that the existence of such consent may be hard to verify at a later date. This concern is increased when obtaining consent over the telephone, although it is still potentially valid. It can be difficult to be sure that the person giving consent is the one who actually has parental responsibility, even when meeting face to face. Over the telephone, there is more uncertainty. For this reason, both trusts and defence lawyers regard written consent as mandatory. For surgery performed on children for cosmetic, social or religious reasons, obtaining consent from both parents is encouraged and is considered to be best practice. A 10-year-old boy may certainly have sufficient capacity to give consent for this procedure, but it is likely that the surgery is being performed at his parents' request, so it may be marginally better to confirm their consent rather than rely exclusively on his.

25. C: Recur after surgery

Inguinal hernias in premature boy neonates have a substantial chance of recurring (in about 5% of cases). Inguinal hernias in children are nearly always indirect, the gut passing through the peritoneal channel made by the processus vaginalis. The direct form of hernia (a bulge through the posterior wall of the inguinal canal) is very rare in the absence of an underlying connective tissue disorder. Spontaneous resolution has been recorded, and would be expected to involve a transient transformation into a hydrocoele. The patent processus would have to close to the point where the entry of gut through the deep ring into the inguinal region was prevented. This would convert the hernia into a hydrocoele, where fluid could still flow into and out of the sac via the narrowed, but still patent, processus. The endpoint of the natural history would see the processus closing completely, leaving evidence of neither a hernia nor a hydrocoele. However, although both these situations are encountered anecdotally, they are relatively rare. If an inguinal hernia becomes incarcerated, it may damage adjacent tissues. The effects of local pressure cause such damage. Pressure on the testicular vessels can cause ischaemia and atrophy of the testis. However, another cause of testicular vessel damage is the herniotomy operation needed to repair the hernia, which may prove to be a very difficult procedure. It may be impossible to identify which mechanism was responsible if testicular atrophy follows hernia incarceration.

Gastroenterology

Mark Beattie

Multiple Choice Questions

1. The following is true of coeliac disease

○ A incidence is 1 in 20,000 in the UK
○ B a negative immunoglobulin A (IgA) endomysial antibody test in a child taking a normal diet excludes the diagnosis
○ C duodenal biopsy is adequate to make the diagnosis
○ D crypt hypertrophy is seen on small bowel biopsy
○ E rice should be excluded from the diet

2. Coeliac disease is associated with

○ A IgA deficiency
○ B herpes stomatitis
○ C human leukocyte antigen (HLA) B8
○ D small bowel malignancy
○ E diabetes mellitus

3. The following is true of Peutz–Jeughers syndrome

○ A it is inherited in an autosomal recessive manner
○ B yellow nails are one of the recognised features
○ C it is pre-malignant
○ D it is associated with peri-oral pigmentation
○ E it is the commonest cause of polyposis in childhood

4. Blind loop syndrome (bacterial overgrowth)

○ A can occur in Crohn's disease
○ B consists of colonisation of the colon with enteric bacteria
○ C leads to excessive vitamin B_{12} absorption
○ D may diminish disaccharidase activity
○ E may lead to steatorrhoea

questions

5. **If a child has abdominal pain and blood in the stools then the following should be considered as part of the differential diagnosis**

    ○ A Meckel's diverticulum
    ○ B *Campylobacter* infection
    ○ C abdominal migraine
    ○ D Crohn's disease
    ○ E mesenteric adenitis

6. **Bloody diarrhoea is characteristic of infection with**

    ○ A *Campylobacter*
    ○ B *Cryptosporidium*
    ○ C *Giardiasis*
    ○ D *Shigella* spp
    ○ E rotavirus

7. **In Gilbert syndrome**

    ○ A conjugated bilirubin is increased
    ○ B the bilirubin level decreases with fasting
    ○ C the jaundice is not detectable clinically
    ○ D kernicterus can occur
    ○ E there are typical histological features on liver biopsy

8. **Long-chain triglyceride absorption requires**

    ○ A intraluminal bile salts
    ○ B trypsin
    ○ C a pH greater than 5
    ○ D an intact jejunum
    ○ E the formation of micelles

9. **In the brush border of the small intestine**

    ○ A lactase hydrolyses lactose into glucose and galactose
    ○ B maltase hydrolyses maltose into glucose and fructose
    ○ C sucrase hydrolyses sucrose into glucose and galactose
    ○ D sucrase hydrolyses sucrose into fructose and galactose
    ○ E galactase hydrolyses lactose into glucose and galactose

10. **The following are absorbed in the terminal ileum**

    ○ A folic acid
    ○ B vitamin B_{12}
    ○ C iron
    ○ D bile acids
    ○ E xylose

11. Chronic active hepatitis can occur following

○ A hepatitis A
○ B hepatitis C
○ C treatment with isoniazid
○ D chlorpromazine therapy
○ E hepatitis B

12. The following are recognised features of Behçet syndrome

○ A non-erosive arthritis
○ B thrombophlebitis
○ C alopecia
○ D meningoencephalitis
○ E resolution of orogenital ulceration with aciclovir

13. Causes of faltering growth include

○ A low birth weight
○ B Duchenne muscular dystrophy
○ C inadequate intake
○ D renal tubular acidosis
○ E pre-term gestation

14. Characteristic features of Crohn's disease include

○ A aphthous mouth ulcers
○ B ankylosing spondylitis
○ C sclerosing cholangitis
○ D raised inflammatory indices
○ E growth retardation

15. Features of ulcerative colitis include

○ A anal fissures
○ B dilated rectum
○ C increased risk of malignancy
○ D granulomatous lesions in the bowel wall
○ E growth failure

16. In a child with glucose galactose malabsorption

○ A lactose is the preferred carbohydrate source
○ B small bowel biopsy is indicated
○ C stool-reducing substances will be negative
○ D inheritance is autosomal dominant
○ E diarrhoea occurs from birth

17. The following is true of of recurrent abdominal pain

- ○ A it affects up to 10% of the school age population
- ○ B it is usually organic
- ○ C it requires further investigation in most cases
- ○ D coeliac disease is a recognised cause
- ○ E it is more common in boys

18. In a child with recurrent abdominal pain an organic cause is suggested by

- ○ A a 3-year history
- ○ B loin pain
- ○ C a family history of migraine
- ○ D raised inflammatory markers
- ○ E diarrhoea

19. *Giardia lamblia*

- ○ A is a protozoal parasite which is infective in the cyst form
- ○ B can cause chronic diarrhoea
- ○ C always requires treatment
- ○ D diagnosis is by serology
- ○ E metronidazole is the antibiotic of first choice

20. Features of Shwachman–Diamond syndrome include

- ○ A abnormal sweat test
- ○ B autosomal recessive inheritance
- ○ C thrombocytopenia
- ○ D tall stature
- ○ E poor response to pancreatic enzyme supplementation

21. Features of portal hypertension include

- ○ A gastric varices
- ○ B thrombocytosis
- ○ C hypoalbuminaemia
- ○ D neutropenia
- ○ E need for anticoagulation

22. Children with cystic fibrosis are at increased risk of

- ○ A intussusception
- ○ B rectal prolapse
- ○ C pancreatitis
- ○ D constipation
- ○ E recurrent abdominal pain of childhood

23. The following statements are true

- ○ A obesity was declared a global epidemic by the World Health Organization (WHO) in 1998
- ○ B there is an increased incidence of type 2 diabetes in children with obesity
- ○ C body mass index = weight/(height)^2
- ○ D 10% of obese children have an underlying physical cause
- ○ E low birth weight is a risk factor

Best of Five Questions

24. **In a child with suspected gastro-oesophageal reflux, which of the following is the MOST useful investigation?**

- A Barium meal
- B Barium swallow
- C pH study
- D Oesophageal biopsy
- E Radionucleotide milk scan

25. **In a child in whom pancreatic insufficiency is suspected and cystic fibrosis has been excluded, the MOST useful investigation would be which of the following?**

- A Stool α_1-antitrypsin
- B Stool chromatography
- C Stool faecal calprotectin
- D Stool faecal elastase
- E Stool microscopy for faecal fats

26. **A girl aged 2 presents with generalised fatigue. Basic investigations show a borderline low haemoglobin, low serum iron, and raised transferrin. MCV (mean cell volume) is 76. She has a mild thrombocytosis. Coeliac screen is negative. Of the five options below, which is the MOST likely cause?**

- A Dietary
- B Occult blood loss
- C Gastro-oesophageal reflux
- D Infection
- E Haemoglobinopathy

27. **In a child referred with suspected peanut allergy, what would the NEXT best step be?**

- A Peanut challenge
- B Advice and dietetic input with regard to peanut exclusion
- C Skin prick test
- D Supply of an epinephrine (adrenaline) pen
- E Ig E radioallergosorbent (RAST) testing

Extended Matching Questions

28. Theme: Abdominal pain

A   Ulcerative colitis
B   Crohn's disease
C   Cystic fibrosis
D   Coeliac disease
E   Gastro-oesophageal reflux
F   Wilm's tumour
G   Hirschsprung disease
H   Constipation
I   Abdominal migraine
J   Diabetes

For each of the following scenarios select the most likely diagnosis from the above list of possible diagnoses. Each option may be used once, more than once, or not at all.

○   1. An 11-year-old girl presents with recurrent abdominal pain over 3 months. She is well in herself but has recently started at secondary school. There is no history of weight loss. She is out of school more than half of the time. She was previously well and there is no relevant family history. Tissue transglutaminase is positive.

○   2. A 14-year-old girl presents with a 6-week history of abdominal pain, bloody diarrhoea and weight loss. Platelet count is raised but other inflammatory markers are normal. Stool culture is negative.

○   3. A 13-year-old boy presents with a 6-month history of recurrent abdominal pain. The pain occurs mostly in the evenings, just before he goes to sleep. He is not missing school. There is a past history of recurrent abdominal pain, although the last time it was a major problem was when he was 11 years. There is an abdominal mass. Basic bloods are normal.

29. Theme: Investigations

A   Hydrogen breath test
B   Stool-reducing substances
C   Duodenal biopsy
D   Carbon-13 urease breath test
E   Serum cholesterol
F   Vitamin E levels
G   Stool chromatography
H   Serology
I   Stool culture
J   Biopsy culture

For the following three conditions select the most appropriate investigation from those listed above. Each option may be used once, more than once, or not at all.

  ◯ 1. Sucrase isomaltase deficiency.
  ◯ 2. *Helicobacter pylori* infection.
  ◯ 3. Abetalipoproteinaemia.

30. Theme: Feeds

A   Normal feed appropriate for age
B   Half-strength milk
C   Lactose-free feed
D   Hydrolysed feed
E   Soya milk
F   Breast milk
G   Oral rehydration solution
H   Fructose-based formula
I   None of the above
J   MCT(medium-chain triglyceride)-based formula

For each of the following clinical scenarios select the most appropriate feed. Each option may be used once, more than once, or not at all.

  ◯ 1. A child with persistent watery diarrhoea after rotavirus infection.
  ◯ 2. A child who develops acute urticaria following the introduction of formula feed.
  ◯ 3. A child admitted with acute gastroenteritis once rehydrated.

answers

1. Coeliac disease

Answers: C D

Prevalence of coeliac disease is 1 in 2000 although this may be an underestimate. The prevalence in Italy is probably nearer to 1 in 300. Intolerance is to gluten which is present in wheat, rye, barley, and oats, although there is some controversy about the exclusion of oats. It normally presents after 6 months of age (i.e. after gluten has been introduced into the diet). Atypical features at presentation are common. IgA anti-endomysial antibody is the most sensitive and specific test in routine use. More recently, tissue transglutaminase is being used which is more sensitive and specific. False negatives occur in children who are IgA-deficient. Diagnosis is by small bowel biopsy. This can be either endoscopic biopsy of the third part of the duodenum or by Crosby capsule biopsy of the proximal jejunum. It is crucial that gluten intake is adequate at the time of the biopsy. Characteristic features on biopsy include sub-total villous atrophy, crypt hypertrophy, intra-epithelial lymphocytes, and a lamina propria plasma cell infiltrate.

2. Coeliac disease

Answers: A C D E

Associations of coeliac disease are with HLA B8, HLA DR7, HLA DR3 and HLA DQw2 with an increased incidence in first degree relatives. There is an increased incidence of small bowel malignancy, especially lymphoma. Coeliac disease is more common in children with IgA deficiency. There is an increased incidence of autoimmune thyroid disease, pernicious anaemia and diabetes mellitus (HLA B8 associations). There is an association with dermatitis herpetiformis. Herpes stomatitis is not a feature.

3. Peutz–Jeghers syndrome

Answers: C D

Peutz–Jeugher syndrome is one of the causes of gastrointestinal polyps. It has autosomal dominant inheritance. Diffuse gastrointestinal hamartomatous polyps in the stomach, small intestine and colon are associated with hyperpigmentation of the buccal mucosa and lips. The syndrome is pre-malignant with an increased risk of gastrointestinal cancer and ovarian tumours.

4. Blind loop syndrome

Answers: A D E

Bacterial overgrowth occurs in the small bowel. Stasis causes bacterial proliferation with the emergence of resistant strains. Repeated courses of antibiotics are a risk factor. Malabsorption results with steatorrhoea and fat-soluble vitamin malabsorption. Disaccharidase activity may be reduced. Diagnosis is by a high index of suspicion, particularly in patients with risk factors such as previous gastrointestinal surgery or short bowel syndrome. Hydrogen breath testing may be useful. Radioisotope-labelled breath testing may also have a role, and barium radiology if obstruction is suspected. Treatment involves appropriate management of the underlying cause. Metronidazole, which is effective orally or intravenously, is the antibiotic of first choice. Probiotics have been used.

5. Abdominal pain with blood in stools

Answers: A B D

It is important to revise the causes of rectal bleeding. Meckel's diverticulum can present with pain and blood per rectum although it usually presents without pain unless there is intussusception. Abdominal pain associated with bloody diarrhoea is however generally indicative of a colitis. Colitis can be infective (as with *Campylobacter*) or non-infective (as with Crohn's disease). Causes of infective and non-infective colitis should be learnt. Mesenteric adenitis and abdominal migraine are both conditions where the diagnosis relies on the absence of systemic features and, in particular, blood per rectum. It is important to remember constipation with fissuring as another cause of pain and blood per rectum. Note the phrase 'be considered' in the question, which implies potential causes and so includes rare causes.

6. Bloody diarrhoea

Answers: A D

Bloody diarrhoea is characteristic of bacterial gastroenteritis when the colon is inflamed. Common bacterial pathogens causing infective colitis include *Campylobacter* (the most common), *Shigella* spp, *Salmonella* spp, enteropathogenic *Escherichia coli*, enterotoxigenic *E. coli* 0157:H7 (rare, but associated with haemolytic uraemic syndrome), *Vibrio cholerae*, and *Yersinia enterocolitica*. It is important also to remember non-infective causes of colitis, such as ulcerative colitis, as part of the differential diagnosis.

7. Gilbert syndrome

Answer: All false

Gilbert syndrome is an unconjugated hyperbilirubinaemia with no evidence of haemolysis. Liver function tests and liver histology are normal. The prevalence is 6%. The condition is more common in boys than in girls.

Inheritance is autosomal dominant with incomplete expression. The pathogenesis is unclear but probably represents a mild functional deficiency of the enzyme uridine diphosphate (UDP) glucuronyl transferase. The clinical picture is of mild fluctuating jaundice (serum bilirubin 30–50 μmol/L) aggravated by infection, exertion and fasting. Of some diagnostic use is the fact that the condition improves with phenobarbitone and worsens with nicotinic acid.

8. Long-chain triglyceride absorption

Answers: A E

It is important to revise the physiology of digestion. Entry of fats into the duodenum causes release of pancreozymin cholecystokinin which stimulates the gall bladder to contract. Hydrolysis of triglycerides occurs. Free fatty acids, glycerol and monoglycerides are emulsified by bile salts to form micelles which arc then absorbed along the brush border of mucosal cells. Short-chain fatty acids enter the portal circulation bound to albumin. Long-chain ones are re-esterified within the mucosal cells into triglycerides, which combine with lesser amounts of protein, phospholipid and cholesterol to create chylomicrons. Chylomicrons enter the lymphatic system and are transported via the thoracic duct to the blood stream.

9. Disaccharidases

Answer: A

Disaccharidases (maltase, sucrase, lactase) in the microvilli hydrolyse oligo- and disaccharides into monosaccharides: maltose into glucose, isomaltose into glucose, sucrose into glucose and fructose, and lactose into glucose and galactose.

10. Terminal ileum absorption

Answers: B D

The sites of absorption are: duodenum and jejunum (fluids, carbohydrates, proteins, fat, iron, calcium, zinc, folate and most vitamins); terminal ileum (vitamin B_{12}, bile salts, vitamin K and vitamin C); colon (water, sodium and fermented carbohydrates).

11. Chronic active hepatitis

Answers: B C E

Chronic active hepatitis refers to inflammation, necrosis and fibrosis that can lead to cirrhosis. The most common causes are hepatitis B, hepatitis C (not hepatitis A) and autoimmune liver disease. Other causes include Wilson's disease, α_1-antitrypsin deficiency, and inflammatory bowel disease (sclerosing cholangitis). Chlorpromazine produces a hypersensitivity response.

answers

12. Behçet syndrome

Answers: A B D

Behçet syndrome is characterised by orogenital ulceration with or without non-erosive arthritis, thrombophlebitis, vascular thromboses or central nervous system abnormalities (including meningoencephalitis). Treatment of orogenital ulceration is often unsatisfactory, although local or systemic steroids may be used acutely. Other drugs that have been used in prophylaxis include azathioprine and thalidomide.

13. Faltering growth

Answers: C D E

Please note the change in terminology: faltering growth is synonymous with failure to thrive. It refers to the failure to gain weight at an adequate rate. It is common in infancy, occurring because a child is in negative energy balance. Low birth weight is a risk factor but not a cause of faltering growth. Duchenne muscular dystrophy usually presents after the child's second birthday and is associated with excess weight gain. Remember that failure to thrive occurs as a consequence of one or more factors of inadequate intake, increased requirements, or excess losses.

14. Crohn's disease

Answers: A D E

The common presenting features of Crohn's disease in childhood are abdominal pain, diarrhoea, weight loss, and impaired linear growth. The diagnosis is made on the basis of clinical symptoms, raised inflammatory indices, and diagnostic tests including barium radiology and colonoscopy with biopsy. Most children have raised inflammatory markers both at presentation and when the disease is active. Ankylosing spondylitis is seen but is not a characteristic feature. Similarly, sclerosing cholangitis is seen in childhood inflammatory bowel disease – but is not a characteristic feature.

15. Ulcerative colitis

Answers: B C E

Peri-anal disease including fissures, abscesses and fistulae are features of Crohn's disease. Ulcerative colitis involves the colonic and rectal mucosa and submucosa. A dilated rectum can be seen in severe disease. Histology is mucosal and submucosal inflammation with goblet cell depletion, cryptitis, and crypt abscesses – but not granulomas, which are a feature of Crohn's disease. Growth failure is a well-recognised feature.

16. Glucose galactose malabsorption

Answer: E

This is a rare autosomal recessively inherited condition characterised by a rapid onset of watery diarrhoea from birth. It responds to withholding glucose (stopping feeds) and relapses on re-introduction. The diagnosis is essentially a clinical one. Reducing substances in the stool will be positive and small bowel biopsy and disaccharide estimation will be normal. Treatment is by using fructose as the main carbohydrate source. Fructose is absorbed by a different mechanism to glucose and galactose.

17. Recurrent abdominal pain

Answers: A D

Recurrent abdominal pain is very common in childhood affecting up to 10% of school-age children. In the majority of cases the aetiology is non-organic. The condition is more common in girls than boys and a family history is common. The pain is usually peri-umbilical and rarely associated with other gastrointestinal symptoms such as diarrhoea, blood per rectum, or weight loss. Abdominal pain accompanied by other symptoms is suggestive of organic pathology. Night pain is suggestive of oesophagitis or peptic ulceration. Diarrhoea with blood per rectum suggests a colitis, and diarrhoea associated with weight loss suggests a malabsorption syndrome. Children with chronic abdominal pain lasting for longer than 3 months should have a basic blood screen including inflammatory markers and coeliac disease serology.

18. Recurrent abdominal pain

Answers: B D E

Recurrent abdominal pain is mostly non-organic. A long history is not a risk factor for organic pathology, being equally a feature in non-organic pain. Loin pain suggests either renal pathology or constipation. A positive family history of migraine is common in children with non-organic abdominal pain in childhood, many of whom go on to suffer from recurrent tension headache as adults. Raised inflammatory markers strongly suggest organic pathology as does diarrhoea, although a common cause for the latter is overflow secondary to constipation. Factors that suggest an organic cause include: age greater than 5 years; constitutional symptoms (fever, weight loss, poor growth, joint symptoms, skin rashes); vomiting (particularly if bile-stained); pain that awakens the child from sleep; pain away from the umbilicus and/or referred to the back or shoulders; urinary symptoms; family history of inflammatory bowel disease or peptic ulcer disease; peri-anal disease; occult or gross blood in the stool; abnormal screening blood tests.

answers

19. *Giardia lamblia*

Answers: A B E

Giardia lamblia is a protozoal parasite which is infective in the cyst form. It also exists in the trophozoite form. It is found in contaminated food and water. Clinical manifestations vary; can be asymptomatic, acute diarrhoeal disease, chronic diarrhoea. Partial villous atrophy is occasionally seen. Diagnosis is by stool examination for cysts or examination of the duodenal aspirate at small bowel biopsy. Treatment is with metronidazole and is often given blind in suspicious cases.

20. Shwachman–Diamond syndrome

Answers: B C

Shwachman–Diamond syndrome is autosomal recessive with an incidence of 1 in 20–200, 000. The main features are pancreatic insufficiency, neutropenia and short stature; other features include metaphyseal dysostosis, mild hepatic dysfunction, increased frequency of infections and further haematological abnormalities (including thrombocytopenia and increased risk of malignancy). Sweat test will be negative but stool faecal elastase as a marker of pancreatic function will be reduced. Formal pancreatic function testing may be necessary. Children respond well to pancreatic supplements.

21. Portal hypertension

Answers: A C D

Clinical features of portal hypertension are splenomegaly; cutaneous porto-systemic shunts (caput medusae – flow from the umbilicus, venous hum above the umbilicus, haemorrhoids); ascites, hypoalbuminaemia, increased incidence of infections; small liver or hepatomegaly; failure to thrive, and reduced muscle bulk. As a consequence of the porto-systemic shunts there is gastrointestinal haemorrhage (oesophageal varices, internal haemorrhoids) and encephalopathy. As a consequence of the large spleen (hypersplenism) there can be thrombocytopenia, anaemia and leukopenia.

22. Cystic fibrosis

Answers: All true

Children with cystic fibrosis, like children with other chronic childhood conditions, are at increased risk of recurrent abdominal pain of childhood (non-organic). There are clearly many stressful and other factors in these children in addition to those seen in healthy children. Gastrointestinal complications of cystic fibrosis can be pancreatic, intestinal or hepatobiliary. Pancreatic complications include insufficiency which occurs in up to 90%; pancreatitis; abnormal glucose tolerance in up to 10% by the second decade; diabetes mellitus). Intestinal complications include meconium ileus, atresias, rectal prolapse, distal obstruction syndrome, and strictures secondary to high-dose pancreatic supplementation (controversial). Hepatobiliary include cholestasis in infancy, fatty liver, focal biliary fibrosis, multilobular cirrhosis, cholelithiasis, or obstruction of the common bile duct.

23. Obesity

Answers: A B C E

Obesity is an important and very topical health care issue. The WHO declared obesity a global epidemic in 1998 with prevalence and severity increasing at alarming rates. There are important short-term and long-term health and social sequelae. Definition is excess body fat, and the body mass index (BMI) should be measured and plotted on an age appropriate chart (overweight > 91st centile; obesity > 98th centile). The aetiology is mainly environmental, reflecting behavioural changes relating to diet and activity. The complications and consequences are of relevance because of the significant effect upon diseases and their presentation, namely: increased incidence of hypertension, hyperlipidaemia and abnormal glucose tolerance in childhood and adolescence; long term increased risk of cardiovascular disease, cerebrovascular disease and type 2 diabetes, osteoarthritis, breast and gastrointestinal malignancy, aggravation of respiratory or rheumatological complaints; increased risk of hepatic steatosis and cholelithiasis; increased risk of psychological and psychosocial problems that persist into adulthood; orthopaedic complications; night hypoventilation, sleep apnoea, and impaired concentration. Most children suffer from simple obesity (99%), that is with no underlying physical cause, and this is the most important part of the initial assessment. Management is to deal with the abnormal fat accumulation which reflects positive energy balance due to excess energy/fat intake and/or decreased energy expenditure (i.e. to switch to negative energy balance by behavioural modification). This is not always easy but methods include increasing exercise, reducing sedentary behaviour and dietary modification. These strategies are time consuming and difficult to implement and such children require considerable support. All practitioners must be aware of and help to deal with this cohort because of the significant short- and long-term impact on morbidity and mortality and so health care needs. Low birth weight is a risk factor for subsequent obesity.

24. C: pH study

Although many children with reflux do not need further investigation, if done, a pH study is the most useful; it is the gold standard for acid reflux, although alkaline reflux will be missed. The strength of the investigation is that it can be done over a 24-hour period and it relates temporally with events (feeds, apnoea). Barium radiology is not particularly sensitive or specific but will pick up anatomical problems such as malrotation or stricture. A nuclear medicine 'milk' scan will assess acid or alkali reflux following a physiological meal. Upper gastrointestinal endoscopy with biopsy will detect oesophagitis but may be negative in the presence of reflux.

25. D: Stool faecal elastase

α_1-Antitrypsin is a serum protein. It is not present in the diet. It has the same molecular weight as albumin. Faecal levels reflect enteric protein loss (protein-losing enteropathy). Chromatography will detect carbohydrate intolerance. Calprotectin is a neutrophil protein, stable in faeces, found in both adults and children to be a simple and non-invasive measure of bowel inflammation. Elastase is a pancreas-specific enzyme which is stable during intestinal transport and is stable in faeces. It is a reliable, indirect marker of pancreatic function although false-positives can occur in short gut and bacterial overgrowth.

26. A: Dietary

The most common cause of iron deficiency anaemia is dietary, involving particularly prolonged or excessive milk feeding. Other causes include chronic blood loss (eg oesophagitis) and malabsorbtion. Dietary sources include cereals, red meat (particularly liver), fresh fruit, and green vegetables. Iron is absorbed from the proximal small bowel. Vitamin C, gastric acid, and protein improve absorption. Deficiency causes hypochromic microcytic anaemia associated with poor appetite and reduced intellectual function. A child with a haemoglobinopathy and iron deficiency would be expected to have a lower mean cell volume (MCV).

27. C: Skin prick test

Peanut and nut allergy are being seen with increasing frequency. It is important to remember that peanuts are a vegetable rather than a true nut. Around 60%–80% of children with peanut allergy are also allergic to other nuts. Reactions vary from mild urticaria to life-threatening anaphylaxis. Skin prick testing is useful, having high sensitivity and specificity. It is important to get the diagnosis right; lots of children have non-specific reactions during childhood and are labelled as peanut allergic. Peanut avoidance is difficult and dietetic support is essential. Even when food labels do not list nuts among the ingredients, contamination may have occurred in trace amounts because of cross contamination from other food production lines. There is some controversy about whether all nuts should be avoided in peanut-allergic patients, and about whether peanut oils should be given. The natural history suggests that children with early onset allergy may grow out of it, although older children with symptomatic reactions are more likely to persist. First-line investigation involves skin prick testing. Active management involves challenge of children whose skin prick tests were negative for peanuts. This is clearly not without risk and needs to be done in an in-patient setting that has facilities for resuscitation.

28. ABDOMINAL PAIN

1.   D – Coeliac disease
The tissue transglutaminase antibody is highly sensitive and specific for coeliac disease. Coeliac serology should be sent on any child with chronic gastrointestinal symptoms.

2.   A – Ulcerative colitis
This could be either Crohn's or ulcerative colitis, but inflammatory markers are almost universally raised in Crohn's disease and so the normal C-reactive protein (CRP) favours ulcerative colitis.

3.   H – Constipation
The presence of a mass, particularly if it will indent on palpation in a child with recurrent abdominal pain, is a pointer to chronic constipation with faecal loading as a potential cause. This is a common cause of a faecal mass. Obviously in such a child there would need to be a low threshold for further investigation, including basic bloods plus or minus plain abdominal X-ray and ultrasound.

29. INVESTIGATIONS

1.   G – Stool chromatography
Sucrase isomaltase deficiency is a defect in carbohydrate digestion with the enzyme required for hydrolysis of sucrose and alpha limit dextrins not present in the small intestine. Symptoms can be very mild. Stools are acidic, but reducing substances are negative as sucrose is a non-reducing sugar and so stool chromatography is required. Management is by removal of sucrose and complex carbohydrate from the diet.

2.   D – Carbon-13 urease breath test
Serology is neither sensitive nor specific. It is difficult to culture the organism. The carbon-13 rapid urease breath test, if positive, is a sensitive and specific indicator of active infection. Histology will show gastritis with organisms present in most cases on specific staining, but this is less sensitive. CLO testing, which is rapid urease testing on biopsy, is both sensitive and specific.

3.   E – Serum cholesterol
Abetalipoproteinaemia is a rare autosomal recessive condition. Pathogenesis is failure of chylomicron formation, with impaired absorption of long-chain fats and fat retention in the enterocyte. Diagnosis is by low serum cholesterol, very low plasma triglyceride level, acanthocytes on examination of the peripheral blood film, and absence of β-lipoprotein in the plasma. Treatment is by substituting medium-chain triglycerides for long-chain triglycerides in the diet.

30. FEEDS

1.   C – Lactose-free feed
This child has probably developed a transient carbohydrate intolerance after infection. This is common in children after rotavirus infection. Treatment is with lactose exclusion until symptoms resolve and then reintroduction of a normal feed after 4–6 weeks.

2.   D – Hydrolysed feed

This child is likely to be allergic to cow's milk protein and will need to be treated with a feed that is free of cow's milk protein. The first choice is a hydrolysate in which the protein is pre-digested. Soya formulae should not be used in infants under 6 months, and in any case there is a significant cross reactivity. The natural history is resolution. Dietetic input is essential as hydrolysed feeds are less palatable than whole-protein feeds and therefore are difficult to give.

3.   A – Normal feed appropriate for age

Standard management of acute gastroenteritis is oral rehydration therapy (if tolerated) to rehydrate, followed by a rapid return to a normal diet once rehydrated. Graded reintroduction of feed or alternative milks is only indicated in complicated gastroenteritis (eg following rotavirus gastroenteritis).

Genetics

Louise C. Wilson

Multiple Choice Questions

1. Examples of X-linked recessive disorders include

- A Becker muscular dystrophy
- B glucose-6-phosphatase deficiency
- C Hunter syndrome (mucopolysaccharidosis type II)
- D Lesch–Nyhan syndrome
- E Rett syndrome

2. In fragile X syndrome

- A boys and girls can be affected
- B the *FMR1* (fragile site mental retardation) pre-mutation can be carried by boys who are unaffected
- C the mutation can be passed from father to son
- D diagnosis is most reliably made by karyotyping for the fragile site
- E all the sons of a mother who is a full-mutation carrier will be affected

3. Congenital myotonic dystrophy

- A is usually seen in the offspring of men with myotonic dystrophy
- B is the most likely outcome in the offspring of an affected female
- C is associated with antenatal polyhydramnios
- D is associated with congenital cataracts
- E is usually associated with learning disability

4. The following is true of cystic fibrosis

- A it can be excluded in a child with no preceding family history of the condition if mutation screening of the *CFTR* (cystic fibrosis transmembrane regulator) is negative
- B it usually presents with meconium ileus
- C it is excluded by negative *IRT* (neonatal immune reactive trypsinogen) screening
- D it causes poor sperm motility in adult men who are affected
- E carrier screening is not usually available for members of the wider family

5. Disorders associated with abnormalities of genomic imprinting include

- ○ A Beckwith–Wiedemann syndrome
- ○ B Williams syndrome
- ○ C Prader–Willi syndrome
- ○ D transient neonatal diabetes
- ○ E Silver–Russell syndrome

6. In neurofibromatosis type 1, features present in the majority of affected individuals by adulthood include

- ○ A at least six café-au-lait patches
- ○ B vestibular schwannomas (acoustic neuromas)
- ○ C flexural freckling
- ○ D plexiform neurofibromas
- ○ E optic glioma

7. The following is true of a child with achondroplasia

- ○ A if both parents are unaffected there is likely to be wrong paternity
- ○ B monitoring for hydrocephalus is unnecessary if neonatal cranial ultrasounds are normal
- ○ C there is an increased risk of obstructive sleep apnoea
- ○ D spinal cord compression is a recognised complication
- ○ E there is likely to be a heterozygous mutation in the *FGFR3* (fibroblast growth factor receptor) gene

8. In autosomal dominant conditions

- ○ A new mutations are common
- ○ B variable expression is common among affected individuals within a family
- ○ C non-penetrance is the term used when an unaffected individual is shown not to have inherited the mutant gene
- ○ D the offspring of an affected person have around a 25% chance of being affected
- ○ E increased severity in successive generations (anticipation) is characteristic

9. Noonan syndrome

- ○ A only occurs in males
- ○ B can be associated with hypertrophic cardiomyopathy
- ○ C can be associated with abnormal blood clotting
- ○ D is always associated with mutations in the *PTPN11* (protein tyrosine kinase, non-receptor type 11) gene
- ○ E is a cause of nuchal oedema on antenatal scans

10. A person with a balanced Robertsonian chromosome translocation

○ A has a translocation involving two acrocentric chromosomes
○ B has a total chromosome complement of 45 instead of 46
○ C has around a 50% chance of having a child with Down syndrome if the translocation involves chromosome 21
○ D is unlikely to have a child with normal chromosomes
○ E is much more likely to have developmental delay than someone with a normal karyotype

11. FISH (fluorescence in-situ hybridisation) testing on a chromosome sample most reliably diagnoses

○ A Williams syndrome
○ B Prader–Willi syndrome
○ C Di George syndrome
○ D translocation Down syndrome
○ E cri-du-chat (cat cry) syndrome

12. Children with chromosome 22q11 deletions

○ A have increased risk of velopharyngeal insufficiency even if their palate is intact
○ B have increased risk of infections because of neutropenia
○ C have increased risk of seronegative arthritis
○ D have increased risk of hypercalcaemia
○ E should be given lymphocyte-depleted blood if they require transfusion

13. Causes of ambiguous genitalia include

○ A Smith–Lemli–Opitz syndrome
○ B a 45 XO Turner karyotype
○ C 21-hydroxylase deficiency in a child with a 46,XY karyotype
○ D 21-hydroxylase deficiency in a child with a 46,XX karyotype
○ E partial androgen insensitivity in a child with a 46,XY karyotype

14. In Williams syndrome

○ A mis-sense mutations in the elastin gene are usually present
○ B there is a characteristic behavioural phenotype
○ C supra-valvular aortic stenosis is the most characteristic cardiac abnormality
○ D renal artery stenosis is a recognised association
○ E calcium supplementation is usually required

15. In Marfan syndrome

- A the diagnosis is routinely made by screening for fibrillin 1 gene mutations
- B clinical evaluation should include examination for musculoskeletal, ocular, cardiac and skin abnormalities
- C dural ectasia is a recognised feature
- D learning difficulties are common
- E an affected person is at 50% risk for having a child with the neonatal form of Marfan syndrome

16. In Duchenne muscular dystrophy

- A the diagnosis is unlikely if no mutations are found on screening for dystrophin gene mutations
- B the mother of an affected boy is almost certainly a carrier
- C there is an increased chance of mental handicap
- D there is an increased risk of cardiomyopathy in adolescence
- E Klinefelter syndrome may mask the clinical findings in a boy carrying the mutation

17. Mosaicism

- A is a feature of McCune–Albright syndrome
- B can result in a skin appearance known as hypomelanosis of Ito
- C that involves cells of the germ-line can result in more than one child with tuberous sclerosis being born to unaffected parents
- D for a karyotypically normal cell-line in a child with Down syndrome can result in a milder phenotype
- E is almost always detectable by examining skin chromosomes

Best of Five Questions

18. In a child with bilateral lens dislocation, mild joint limitation and learning disability, the MOST likely diagnosis is which of the following?

- A Stickler syndrome
- B Marfan syndrome
- C Ehlers–Danlos syndrome
- D Homocystinuria
- E Benign familial joint hypermobility

19. The normal sister of a boy with Tay–Sachs disease has asked for her risk of being a carrier for the condition. What is the MOST appropriate answer?

- A 100%
- B 66%
- C 50%
- D 33%
- E 25%

20. A Turkish couple are concerned about their offspring risks, given that they are first cousins, although they have no family history of any genetic disorder. Which of the following would be the MOST appropriate testing to offer them?

- A Carrier testing for cystic fibrosis
- B Amniocentesis for chromosomes testing
- C Carrier testing for Gaucher disease
- D Karyotyping on blood
- E Carrier testing for haemoglobinopathies

21. **The mother of a boy with Duchenne muscular dystrophy tells you that her brother was similarly affected and died in his teenage years. She has a sister who is pregnant and they want to know the risk of this sister having an affected boy. Which is the CLOSEST answer from the list below?**

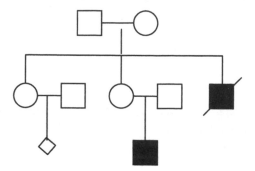

- A 66%
- B 50%
- C 33%
- D 25%
- E 12.5%

22. **A 22-year-old woman who is pregnant tells you she had a sister who died as a baby from a severe atrioventricular septal defect associated with Down syndrome. She has no further information but is concerned about her own risk for having a baby with Down syndrome. The MOST appropriate course of action is which of the following?**

- A To check her chromosomes and proceed with routine maternal serum screening and anomaly scanning if they are normal
- B To check her chromosomes and proceed with routine maternal serum screening and anomaly scanning if they show she carries a Robertsonian translocation between chromosomes 14 and 21
- C To offer chorionic villus sampling for chromosomes at 11 weeks gestation
- D To offer amniocentesis testing for chromosomes at 16 weeks gestation
- E To offer detailed cardiac scanning at 22 weeks gestation

23. **A child has severe neonatal hypotonia. Which of the following is LEAST likely to be the underlying diagnosis?**

- A Spinal muscular atrophy
- B Prader–Willi syndrome
- C Congenital myotonic dystrophy
- D Nemaline myopathy
- E Duchenne muscular dystrophy

24. **A man who has a child with spinal muscular atrophy (SMA) from a previous relationship would like to know his risk of having an affected child with his new unrelated partner who has no family history of any genetic disorder. The background population carrier risk for SMA is 1 in 40. Which of the following BEST represents their risk of having an affected child?**

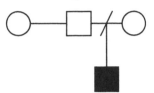

- A 1 in 4
- B 1 in 160
- C 1 in 240
- D 1 in 320
- E 1 in 6400

25. **A 26-year-old man presented with a spinal schwannoma following which he was found to meet the diagnostic criteria for neurofibromatosis type I. He was concerned to know whether his 6-year-old son had inherited the condition. The MOST appropriate first course of action is which of the following?**

- A Collect DNA from the son for screening for mutations in the neurofibromin (*NF1*) gene
- B Arrange magnetic resonance imaging (MRI) of the child's brain and spine
- C Examine the child for café-au-lait patches
- D Arrange an ophthalmology opinion for Lisch nodules and optic glioma
- E Check the child's paternity

26. **In a child with disproportionate short stature the investigation MOST likely to be helpful diagnostically is which of the following?**

- A Mutation testing for achondroplasia
- B Endocrine testing for growth hormone levels and pituitary function
- C A skeletal survey
- D Examination of both parents
- E Assessment of sitting and standing heights and arm span

Extended Matching Questions

27. Theme: Cardiac complications

A   Dilated cardiomyopathy
B   Hypertrophic cardiomyopathy
C   Aortic coarctation
D   Aortic dissection
E   Aortic incompetence
F   Interrupted aortic arch
G   Atrial fibrillation
H   Heart block
I   Pulmonary stenosis
J   Tricuspid regurgitation

For each of the following conditions, select the most common cardiac complication from the list above. Each option may be used once, more than once, or not at all.

   ○   1. Myotonic dystrophy.
   ○   2. Becker muscular dystrophy.
   ○   3. Noonan syndrome.

28. Theme: Conditions that are more common in certain populations

A   Ashkenazi Jewish
B   Mediterranean
C   Afro-Caribbean
D   North European
E   Australian
F   Chinese
G   South African

From the list above, select the population in whom the following conditions are most prevalent. Each option may be used once, more than once, or not at all.

   ○   1. Coeliac disease.
   ○   2. Breast and ovarian cancer.
   ○   3. Variegate porphyria.

29. Theme: Karyotypes

A   45,X
B   45,Y
C   46,XX
D   46,XY
E   47,XXY
F   47,XXX
G   47,XYY
H   45,XY,t(14;21)
I   46,XX,t(14;21)
J   46,XX,t(7;20)

For each of the following conditions select the appropriate karyotype from the list above. Each option may be used once, more than once, or not at all.

○   1. A normal reciprocal translocation carrier.
○   2. A girl with Christmas disease (haemophilia B).
○   3. A boy with Noonan syndrome.

questions

answers

1. X-linked recessive disorders

Answers: A C D

Becker muscular dystrophy results from mutations in the dystrophin gene which usually result in some preservation of dystrophin protein function and hence a milder phenotype than Duchenne muscular dystrophy. In both, female heterozygotes (carriers) frequently have elevated creatine kinase levels, and around 5–10% manifest some mild weakness and/or calf hypertrophy. In both there is some risk (probably around 15%, though estimates vary) of dilated cardiomyopathy in the female carriers, regardless of whether they have other symptoms. Glucose-6-phosphatase deficiency (GSD I) is autosomal recessive. Glucose-6-phosphate dehydrogenase deficiency (favism) is X-linked, so they can be confused. Hunter syndrome (MPS II) is the only mucopolysaccharidosis that is not autosomal recessive. Although the gene for Rett syndrome (*MECP2*) is X-linked, females with mutations almost always manifest, while male conceptions with Rett mutations are not usually viable. This is typical of an X-linked dominant condition.

2. Fragile X syndrome

Answers: A B

Boys with the *FMR1* full mutation are always affected (unless they have coincidental Klinefelter syndrome). Girls with the full mutation have around a 50% chance of showing significant learning disability or behavioural features. The sons of a woman with full mutation have a 50% chance of inheriting a normal X chromosome, in which case they would be unaffected. There is also a 50% chance they would inherit the full mutation (which rarely contracts in size) and so be affected. Pre-mutation carriers of either sex are not affected. A man passes on his Y chromosome to all his sons. He passes his X chromosome to all his daughters, but the pre-mutation does not expand when transmitted through a male, which means that all his daughters will be pre-mutation carriers. In the past, testing was cytogenetic and required culturing of lymphocytes in folate-deficient media to reveal the fragile site. However, this resulted in false-negatives. Modern testing is by molecular genetic analysis to assess the size of the repeat expansion, which is far more reliable.

3. Congenital myotonic dystrophy

Answers: C E

Myotonic dystrophy is an autosomal dominant condition caused by a triplet repeat expansion mutation in the *DMPK* (dystrophia myotonica protein kinase) gene. Broadly, the larger the expansion the earlier the onset of symptoms. The expansion is at greatest risk of further expansion when transmitted through a female and this accounts for the observed tendency to increasing severity in successive generations, known as anticipation. Expansion of the mutation to the size associated with congenital onset is very rare when passed through a male. Men who themselves had a congenital onset rarely reproduce. For affected women, there is a 50% chance that they will pass on the mutant allele, which could remain stable or only enlarge by a small amount. The likelihood of it enlarging sufficiently to cause the congenital form depends to some extent on the size of the expansion in the mother and this roughly correlates with the age at onset of symptoms in the mother. Overall the risk of a congenitally affected offspring will be less than 50%. Congenital myotonic dystrophy is associated with polyhydramnios, reduced fetal movements, talipes, neonatal hypotonia, facial diplegia, thin ribs, and poor respiratory effort. Clinical myotonia is often absent early on. Cataracts are a feature of myotonic dystrophy in later life but not at birth. The congenital onset form is associated with significant learning disability.

4. Cystic fibrosis

Answer: All false

In North European Caucasians, current screening detects around 90% of *CFTR* mutations. That means in about 18% of affected children only one mutation will be detected, and in approximately 1% neither mutation will be detected. In other populations, the detection rate is lower (for Turkish the rate is about 50% and for Asians about 40%) which means that only one mutation or no mutation will be found in a significant proportion of affected patients, although the absolute incidence in these populations is lower. All first-degree relatives of people with cystic fibrosis should be offered carrier screening. In turn the relatives of individuals found to be carriers should be offered screening. This is known as cascade screening. In some health regions, neonatal *IRT* screening is offered. A positive *IRT* test is not diagnostic of cystic fibrosis but warrants further investigation, as the specificity of *IRT* screening is low. *IRT* testing is thought to detect around 90%, at most, of babies with classical cystic fibrosis. Meconium ileus occurs in around 10–15% of patients with cystic fibrosis. Cystic fibrosis is associated with male infertility as a result of azoospermia and/or oligozoospermia secondary to congenital bilateral absence of the vas deferens.

5. Abnormalities of genomic imprinting

Answers: A C D E

Imprinted genes are those for which the parental origin determines the degree to which they are expressed. Imprinting can involve exclusive expression of one parental allele, or relatively greater expression from one allele compared to another. The pattern of parental expression is consistent across all normal individuals. Imprinting of some genes is tissue specific (that is, it can only be detected in certain tissues). Beckwith–Wiedemann syndrome results from abnormal imprinting of the *IGF2/H19/KVLQT1/p57kip (CDKN1C)* gene cluster on chromosome 11p15, although there are several different underlying molecular mechanisms. Prader–Willi syndrome results from absence of a paternal contribution for genes on chromosome 15q11–13. In around 70% it is due to a deletion on the paternal-derived chromosome 15 while in about 30% it is due to maternal uni-parental disomy for chromosome 15 (where both copies of chromosome 15 are maternally derived with no paternal contribution). Transient neonatal diabetes results from abnormal imprinting of a gene(s) on distal chromosome 6q. Most patients have been found to have paternal uni-parental disomy for the region or paternal duplications. Around 15% of patients with Silver–Russell syndrome have maternal uni-parental disomy for chromosome 7. In the remainder, the molecular mechanism is not yet clear.

6. Neurofibromatosis type 1

Answers: A C

Six or more café-au-lait patches are usually present by 4 years of age. Freckling in the axillae and inguinal regions is usually present by adulthood. Large plexiform neurofibromas occur in 5–10% but if the smaller less cosmetically significant ones are included they are present in around 30% of patients with neurofibromatosis type 1. Cranial magnetic resonance scans show optic glioma in around 15%, but clinically significant optic glioma occurs in only about 2%. Acoustic neuromas are a major feature of neurofibromatosis type 2, but not type 1.

7. Achondroplasia

Answers: C D E

This is an example of an autosomal dominant condition with a high new mutation rate (around 80%). Almost all patients with achondroplasia have the same mutation in the *FGFR3* gene. Children with achondroplasia have relatively large heads and separate growth charts are available for them. However, they are at risk for developing hydrocephalus in the first 2 years and should be monitored closely for rapidly increasing head circumference and signs of hydrocephalus throughout this period. The skull base and foramen magnum are small, giving rise to an increased risk of brainstem and cervical cord compression. In addition, the vertebral pedicles are short, which can result in spinal stenosis later. Thoracolumbar gibbus is associated with unsupported sitting early on, and prominent lumbar lordosis is common in older children. Sleep studies should be considered where the children have noisy breathing or intermittent breathing, marked retraction, or snoring, particularly if their developmental milestones are lagging.

8. Autosomal dominant conditions

Answers: A B

Broadly, new autosomal dominant mutations tend to be more common with increasing paternal age, in contrast to chromosomal non-disjunction such as trisomy 21 which is more common with increasing maternal age. Offspring have a 50% chance of inheriting the mutant gene and hence the condition. Variable expression is a term used to describe differences in the severity of particular features of a condition from one affected individual to another. Non-penetrance is a term used when individuals who are known to carry the mutant gene show no clinical features. Anticipation is only a characteristic of certain autosomal dominant conditions where the mutation mechanism is the expansion of an unstable trinucleotide repeat (as in myotonic dystrophy or Huntington's disease).

9. Noonan syndrome

Answers: B C E

Noonan syndrome is an autosomal dominant condition which affects both sexes. Only around 50% have a mutation in the *PTPN11* gene on chromosome 12. In the remainder, the causative gene is not known. In many centres the fetus is screened by ultrasound for increased nuchal oedema at 12 weeks' gestation. The most common causes include trisomy 21, Turner syndrome, congenital infection, severe fetal anaemia, and severe cardiac malformations, but Noonan syndrome is also a recognised cause. The most frequent cardiac abnormality is pulmonary stenosis, often associated with a dysplastic valve. Other well-recognised cardiac abnormalities are hypertrophic cardiomyopathy and septal defects. Feeding difficulties are common. The condition is associated with abnormal clotting.

10. Balanced Robertsonian chromosome translocation

Answers: A B

Acrocentric chromosomes have their centromere at one end so that the short (p) arm does not carry any functional genes. A Robertsonian translocation results from the fusion of two acrocentric chromosomes at (or adjacent to) the centromere. The acrocentric chromosomes are 13, 14, 15, 21 and 22. The process of fusion at (or adjacent to) the centromeres of acrocentric chromosomes does not disrupt any genes and is not usually associated with

answers

any phenotypic abnormality. The fused chromosomes are counted as one, and so there are 45 chromosomes. The translocation carrier also has a normal copy of each of the chromosomes involved in the translocation which they can pass on. In fact, the two most likely outcomes in the offspring of a balanced Robertsonian translocation carrier are that they have normal chromosomes or a balanced translocation like the parent. The observed risk of Down syndrome is 10–15% for a female and 2–3% for a male carrying a Robertsonian translocation involving chromosome 21.

11. FISH testing

Answers: A C E

FISH testing is used to detect sub-microscopic chromosome deletions (microdeletions). Patients with Williams syndrome have deletions which encompass the elastin gene and adjacent genes, Di George syndrome results from 22q11 deletions, and cri-du-chat results from deletions of chromosome 5p, which may be visible on standard microscopy but may be sub-microscopic (therefore it is best tested for by FISH). Although FISH testing will detect patients with Prader–Willi who have a deletion (around 70%) it does not detect the 30% of patients with uni-parental disomy. Molecular genetic (DNA-based) testing is now used for Prader-Willi which screens for both. In translocation Down syndrome, the translocation is best seen on routine karyotyping.

12. Chromosome 22q11 deletions

Answers: A C E

22q11 deletions may manifest as nasal regurgitation of fluids or a nasal sounding voice due to nasal escape secondary to incomplete closing off of the nasopharynx by the palate. The immune abnormalities are secondary to T lymphocyte deficits, and these patients, therefore, should be given lymphocyte-depleted blood. Increased risk of seronegative arthritis is an observation, but the basis is not really clear. There is an increased risk of hypocalcaemia.

13 Ambiguous genitalia

Answers: A D E

Smith–Lemli–Opitz syndrome is a rare autosomal recessive disorder of cholesterol biosynthesis which is a cause of ambiguous (under-masculinised) genitalia in boys. It is diagnosed by finding raised levels of 7–dehydrocholesterol in blood. Genital ambiguity is only associated with Turner syndrome where there is mosaicism for a Y chromosome containing cell line. Chromosomal males with 21-hydroxylase deficiency will appear to be normal boys at birth, whereas chromosomal females may present with masculinised genitalia. Where there is complete androgen insensitivity, chromosomal males will appear to be female, but where the androgen insensitivity is partial there will be some incomplete masculinisation.

14. Williams syndrome

Answers: B C D

Patients with Williams syndrome have deletions encompassing the elastin gene and adjacent (contiguous) genes. Point mutations in the elastin gene cause isolated supra-valvular aortic stenosis. Children have significant cognitive impairment (particularly visual–motor integration) and attention deficit but relatively spared language abilities together with a sociable personality resulting in a characteristic behavioural picture known as a cocktail-party manner. Supra-valvular aortic stenosis is the most characteristic cardiac defect. Others which have been associated include abnormalities of the aortic valve, pulmonary or mitral valves and septal defects. Renal artery stenosis is also a recognised feature. They are at risk of hypercalcaemia in early childhood.

15. Marfan syndrome

Answers: B C

The fibrillin gene is very large and the mutations tend to be family-specific and mutation detection rates tend to be low. For some sequence changes it can be difficult to distinguish which are mutations and which are harmless polymorphisms. As a result, diagnosis is usually based on clinical findings. In a patient with no family history of the condition, formal diagnosis requires major abnormalities in at least two different organ systems (includes skeletal, ocular, cardiovascular, and dural ectasia) and involvement of a third (those mentioned above and the pulmonary system and skin). Where found, dural ectasia is a recognised major criterion. However, it is not currently routinely screened for in the diagnostic evaluation for Marfan syndrome. Intelligence is usually normal. Neonatal Marfan syndrome is a particularly severe form of the condition which is usually fatal in the neonatal period. It is associated with particularly deleterious fibrillin mutations, which have arisen de novo as affected individuals with these mutations do not survive to adulthood. Adults with Marfan syndrome are at 50% risk for passing on to their child the same form of the condition as their own. However, they are not at increased risk for having a child with the neonatal form.

16. Duchenne muscular dystrophy

Answers: C D E

Mutations are currently found in only 66% of males who have a diagnosis of Duchenne muscular dystrophy confirmed by dystrophin immunostaining on muscle. Around one-third (33%) of affected males have a new mutation. Around 30% of boys with Duchenne muscular dystrophy have learning disability. There is an increased risk of dilated cardiomyopathy. Males with Klinefelter syndrome have an XXY sex chromosome pattern and randomly inactivate one of their X chromosomes by lyonisation. Thus, like females they are unlikely to manifest symptoms unless they happen to lyonise unfavourably.

17. Mosaicism

Answers: A B C D

Mosaicism can occur at a single gene or whole chromosome level. It can only be detected cytogenetically if it involves whole chromosomes, which is only the case in a minority. Where present it may be more easily detected in skin, sometimes because the abnormal cells are selected against in blood. New autosomal dominant or X-linked mutations can arise in progenitor cells of the eggs or sperm. They will not be detectable in lymphocyte DNA from the individual. Thus an individual who has one child with a detectable mutation can have a second child with the same mutation despite not themselves having the mutation in other tissues such as blood. This is known as germ-line mosaicism and is important to consider when counselling for autosomal dominant or X-linked disorders. McCune–Albright syndrome is the triad of endocrine hyperfunction, café-au-lait pigmentation and polyostotic fibrous dysplasia. It results from mosaicism for activating mutations in the gene for the alpha subunit of G_s, a heterotrimeric G-protein involved in signal transduction for a number of hormones which act on cell-surface receptors including parathyroid hormone, thyroid stimulating hormone, luteinising hormone and adrenocorticotrophic hormone. Hypomelanosis of Ito is characterised by streaky hypopigmented patches following Blaschko's lines. These run circumferentially around the trunk and longitudinally along the limbs and are believed to represent the lines of migration of clones of epithelial cells. It is an indicator of mosaicism at some level. Around 3% of patients with Down syndrome have mosaicism and usually the associated phenotype is milder.

18. D. Homocystinuria

Marfan syndrome causes lens dislocation, but joints are lax and there is not usually any learning disability.

19. B: 66%

This is an autosomal recessive condition. To have an affected brother, both her parents must be carriers. In each pregnancy her parents had a 1 in 4 chance of having an affected child; a 2 in 4 chance of having a carrier; and a 1 in 4 chance of having an unaffected child who is not a carrier. Given that the sister of the affected boy is unaffected, the first possibility can be eliminated giving a 2 in 3 (66%) chance that she is a carrier.

20. E: Carrier testing for haemoglobinopathies

The autosomal recessive condition for which they are at greatest risk and for which carrier testing is available is β-thalassaemia. Turkish people are not a population with a high carrier risk for cystic fibrosis and the current mutation detection rate in the population is quite low, at around 50% (compared to 90% and 95% in the North European Caucasian and Ashkenazi Jewish populations, respectively). Gaucher disease is common in the Ashkenazi Jewish population but not in Turkish people. The married cousins are at no increased risk for chromosomal abnormalities due to their consanguinity.

21. E: 12.5%

The mother has an affected son and a brother with Duchenne muscular dystrophy which means she is an obligate carrier, as is her own mother. Her sister therefore has a 50% (1 in 2) chance of being a carrier. A female carrier for Duchenne muscular dystrophy has a 25% (1 in 4) chance of an affected son. Overall, then, the sisters risk for having an affected boy is 1 in 8 or 12.5% ($\frac{1}{2} \times \frac{1}{4}$).

22. A: Check her chromosomes and proceed with routine maternal serum screening and anomaly scanning if they are normal

It is most likely that her sister had straightforward trisomy 21. However, the small possibility that it was translocation Down syndrome cannot be excluded, so her chromosomes should be checked. If they are normal, then she is not at any significantly increased risk compared with background risk, and only routine screening is appropriate. If found to carry a Robertsonian translocation involving chromosome 21 then she should be offered fetal karyotyping by chorionic villus sampling or amniocentesis. It is not appropriate to offer invasive testing by chorionic villus sampling or amniocentesis if she is at no increased risk. The atrioventricular septal defect is very likely to be related to the Down syndrome and she is unlikely to be at any increased risk for having a child with a cardiac abnormality from any other cause.

23. E: Duchenne muscular dystrophy

Duchenne muscular dystrophy is not associated with neonatal hypotonia whereas all the others are.

24. B: 1 in 160

If he has had an affected child he can be assumed to be a carrier for SMA. The chance his partner is a carrier is 1 in 40. If they are both carriers, their risk for an affected child is 1 in 4. Overall, therefore, their risk is 1 in 160 ($1 \times \frac{1}{40} \times \frac{1}{4}$).

25. C: Examine the child for café-au-lait patches

The diagnosis of NF1 is still a clinical one. By the age of 4 years, the majority of affected children have six or more café-au-lait patches. Only a minority have an optic glioma on MRI scanning (15%) of which only a small proportion cause symptoms. Lisch nodules are often not present in early childhood. Only a few have spinal or intracranial tumours. Molecular testing is becoming available but the mutation detection rate is not 100%.

26. C: A skeletal survey

Although achondroplasia is a common cause of disproportionate short stature it is not the only one. It can be diagnosed reliably by skeletal survey as can many other causes. Growth hormone deficiency is not associated with disproportionate short stature. The parents could easily be normal if the condition was a new mutation, autosomal dominant or autosomal recessive. Measuring sitting and standing heights and arm span will confirm the disproportion, but this is unlikely to be helpful otherwise.

27. CARDIAC COMPLICATIONS

1.   H – Heart block
Conduction defects are common in adults with myotonic dystrophy and can lead to arrhythmias or sudden death. Affected adults should have their electrocardiogram checked with intervention as and when appropriate.

2.   A – Dilated cardiomyopathy
Dystrophin is expressed in cardiac as well as skeletal muscle and dilated cardiomyopathy is a feature of both Duchenne and Becker muscular dystrophies, and occurs in a small proportion of female carriers, for which they are offered cardiac screening. In some rare families, dystrophin mutations have been associated with an X-linked form of cardiomyopathy in the absence of any symptomatic skeletal muscle weakness.

3.   I – Pulmonary stenosis
The most frequent cardiac abnormality in Noonan syndrome is pulmonary stenosis, often associated with a dysplastic valve. Other well-recognised cardiac abnormalities are hypertrophic cardiomyopathy and septal defects.

28. CONDITIONS THAT ARE MORE COMMON IN CERTAIN POPULATIONS

1.   D – North European
Coeliac disease is a multifactorial disease to which there is a genetically determined susceptibility. It is particularly common in the North European, North American and Finnish populations.

2.   A – Ashkenazi Jewish
There are a small number of autosomal dominant mutations in the *BRCA1* and *BRCA2* genes which are particularly common in the Ashkenazi Jewish population, presumably due to a founder effect, and predispose to breast and ovarian cancer.

answers

3. G – South African

Around 1 in 350 South Africans have autosomal dominant variegate porphyria which can be associated with photosensitivity as well as neurovisceral disturbances. Symptoms before puberty are unusual.

29. KARYOTYPES

1. J – 46,XX,t(7;20)

In contrast to chromosomes 13, 14, 15, 21 and 22, neither chromosomes 7 nor 20 are acrocentric so this translocation must be a reciprocal one where a segment of chromosomes 7 and 20 have been exchanged. This means that in addition to the normal copies of chromosome 7 and 20, there is a 7 with a piece of chromosome 20 replacing part of its length, and a 20 with the corresponding piece of 7 attached. This leaves 46 chromosomes in total in a balanced reciprocal translocation carrier.

2. A – 45,X

The most likely explanation for a female fully manifesting an X-linked disease is that she has Turner syndrome. The other possibility, but a less likely one, is that she has normal chromosomes but has unfavourably skewed X chromosome inactivation.

3. D – 46,XY

Noonan syndrome is not associated with any karyotypic (chromosomal) abnormality.

Haematology and oncology

Michael Capra

Multiple Choice Questions

1. The following is true of iron deficiency anaemia

- A it is the commonest cause of a microcytic hypochromic anaemia in infancy
- B serum transferrin is the most reliable indicator, other than a bone marrow aspiration, of total iron stores
- C it commonly presents from 2 months of age upwards in a term infant
- D the ratio of the mean cell volume (MCV) to the red blood cell count is useful in differentiation from thalassaemia
- E decreased T cell function and cell-mediated immunity is reported

2. With respect to hereditary haemolytic anaemia

- A hereditary spherocytosis is the commonest hereditary haemolytic anaemia in Northern Europe
- B hereditary spherocytosis is confirmed by the presence of spherocytes on the blood smear and by the chromosome fragility test
- C glucose-6-phosphate dehydrogenase (G6PD) deficiency and pyruvate kinase deficiency are inherited in an autosomal recessive manner
- D glucose-6-phosphate dehydrogenase deficiency is confirmed by assaying the red cell G6PD enzyme
- E the Embden–Meyerhof pathway is unable to function in a red cell that is deficient in G6PD

3. The following is true of aplastic anaemia

- A congenital aplastic anaemia is more common than the acquired form
- B Fanconi's anaemia is the commonest cause
- C age-related anaemia is a prerequisite for the diagnosis to be confirmed
- D erythropoietin is an effective treatment in the majority of cases
- E allogeneic bone marrow transplantation is a recognised treatment option

4. Regarding autoimmune haemolytic anaemia (AIHA)

○ A the direct Coombs test will be positive
○ B it is frequently due to an intercurrent viral infection in children
○ C spherocytes are commonly seen on the blood smear.
○ D AIHA is divided into warm and cold types depending on whether the patient is febrile or afebrile
○ E it is often associated with connective tissue disorders in the adolescent

5. The following is true of the ABO blood grouping system

○ A children with group A blood type have naturally occurring anti-A antibodies
○ B children with group O blood type have no naturally occurring antibodies
○ C antibodies directed against red cell antigens are present at birth
○ D the majority of children in the UK will have either type O or A blood groups
○ E the critical blood transfusion principle is for transfused blood not to contain red cells that the recipient's antibodies will react with

6. Red cell physiology

○ A erythropoeitin is produced predominantly by endothelial cells, in response to a reduction of the partial pressure of oxygen in the blood stream
○ B vitamin C (ascorbate) is a coenzyme required in the initial stage of haem synthesis
○ C the mitochondria and ribosomes within the erythroblast produce haem and globin, respectively
○ D a molecule of haemoglobin is comprised of four globin chains attached to their own haem moiety
○ E the red cell generates its own energy by metabolizing glucose only

7. Regarding leukocytes

○ A eosinophils play a role in the defense against parasites
○ B mast cells are derived from basophils
○ C once migrated into the tissue, a neutrophil is called a phagocyte
○ D lymphocytes contain myeloperoxidase
○ E band cells are immature neutrophils

8. von Willebrand disease (vWD)

○ A is caused by a qualitative or quantitative deficiency of von Willebrand factor
○ B the resulting bleeding disorder in vWD is characterized by petechiae
○ C the platelet count is normal
○ D the ristocetin co-factor activity will be decreased
○ E is inherited in an X-linked recessive pattern

9. In neonatal alloimmune thrombocytopenia (NAIT)

- ○ A the most commonly occurring human platelet antigen is HPA-1a
- ○ B the father needs to be HPA negative and the mother positive for the same HPA for alloimmune neonatal thrombocytopenia to develop
- ○ C the first-born child of genetically predisposed parents is commonly involved
- ○ D the thrombocytopenia becomes evident after approximately 5 days of life
- ○ E treatment includes antenatal periumbilical transfusions of maternal donated platelets

10. Blood products

- ○ A fresh frozen plasma contains all coagulation factors and complement
- ○ B cryoprecipitate contains fibrinogen and factor VIII
- ○ C fresh frozen plasma and platelets should be ABO compatible with recipient
- ○ D 1 unit of random donor platelets per 10 kg bodyweight raises platelet count by 10–20 × 10⁹/L
- ○ E the recommended volume for a fresh frozen plasma infusion is 10 ml/kg

11. Regarding coagulation

- ○ A all clotting factors are synthesized in the liver
- ○ B factor VIII is synthesized by hepatocytes and by endothelial cells
- ○ C factor XIII deficiency does not prolong the INR (international normalised ratio) nor the APTT (activated partial thromboplastin time)
- ○ D an isolated factor VII deficiency elevates the APTT only
- ○ E an isolated factor II deficiency results in prolonged APTT, thrombin time (TT) and INR

12. Leukaemia in childhood

- ○ A the majority of leukaemias in childhood are classified as acute
- ○ B chronic lymphocytic leukaemia does not occur in childhood
- ○ C acute lymphoblastic leukaemia (ALL) accounts for 95% of all acute leukaemias
- ○ D the majority of ALL cases are of T cell origin
- ○ E the majority of acute myeloid leukaemia (AML) cases are of B cell origin

13. Regarding the incidence and epidemiology of cancer in children

- ○ A the incidence of childhood cancer in the UK is 1 in 6000 children
- ○ B neuroblastoma is the most commonly occurring solid tumour
- ○ C leukaemia together with lymphoma account for nearly 50% of all cases of malignancy
- ○ D the most common brain tumour is a medulloblastoma
- ○ E boys and girls are equally affected by childhood cancer

14. Poor prognostic signs in acute lymphoblastic leukaemia include

- A the presence of the Philadelphia chromosome (t9:22)
- B age over 10 years at diagnosis
- C age less than 4 years at diagnosis
- D presenting white cell count of greater than 50×10^9/L
- E central nervous system disease

15. In acute myeloid leukaemia (AML)

- A the treatment for AML comprises a 2–3 year chemotherapy regimen
- B erythroblastic leukaemia is one of the subtypes of AML
- C the most common subtype of AML is of B cell origin
- D 5-year survival is 50%
- E secondary AML resulting from previously administered chemotherapy carries an inferior prognosis relative to primary AML

16. The following is true of tumour lysis syndrome (TLS)

- A the two most common malignancies associated with TLS are acute myeloid leukaemia (AML) and B cell non-Hodgkin's lymphoma (NHL)
- B the cause of acute renal failure in TLS is usually due to the precipitation of uric acid and phosphate crystals into the kidney
- C hyperphosphataemia, hypercalcaemia and hyperkalaemia are the commonly observed electrolyte imbalances
- D hyperhydration remains a key element in the prevention of TLS
- E allopurinol is effective in preventing TLS by increasing the solubility of uric acid

17. Causes of an elevated α-fetoprotein (AFP) include

- A ataxia telangiectasia
- B hepatitis
- C hepatoblastoma or hepatocellular carcinoma
- D germ cell tumour, of yolk sac origin
- E Beckwith–Wiedemann syndrome

18. Chemotherapeutic agents

- A vincristine is neurotoxic, potentially resulting in ptosis, peripheral neuropathy or vocal cord paralysis
- B Prednisone is a potent cytotoxic agent
- C asparaginase has the potential to cause a bleeding diathesis or a prothrombotic state
- D daunomycin, an anthracycline agent, is cardiotoxic
- E methotrexate is administered via the oral, intravenous or intrathecal route

19. Regarding the use of radiotherapy in children

○ A the standing height rather than the sitting height of a child may be limited by craniospinal irradiation

○ B inflammable anaesthetic gases are contraindicated when anaesthetising a child for radiotherapy

○ C due to the potential devastating effects of radiotherapy on the developing brain, cranial radiotherapy is contraindicated in children under the age of 7 years

○ D to allow sufficient healing, at least 6 months must have elapsed before administering further radiotherapy to an area that has already received the maximal tolerated dose of radiotherapy

○ E radiotherapy-induced hypothyroidism is a transient phenomenon while radiotherapy-induced growth hormone deficiency is permanent

20. Chemotherapy-induced febrile neutropenic episodes

○ A an absolute neutrophil count of $< 1.5 \times 10^9/L$ and an oral temperature $> 38°C$ are the diagnostic criteria for a febrile neutropenic episode

○ B a child who is neutropenic and who becomes febrile should be treated as a "medical emergency"

○ C administration of broad-spectrum intravenous antibiotics, following a blood culture being drawn, is the recommended initial treatment

○ D if the fever persists for longer than 5 days, investigation and treatment of an underlying fungal aetiology is recommended

○ E paracetamol is the antipyretic of choice in a neutropenic child

Best of Five Questions

21. **A 20-month-old boy presents to you, an inner city practicing paediatrician, with pallor and a cough. He is the first-born child of healthy Asian parents who are distantly related. His younger sister, aged 6 months, is well and thriving. His diet consists of cows' milk, fortified cereal and occasionally vegetables and red meat. Examination apart from pallor is unremarkable. His height and weight are on the 20th percentile. The following haematological parameters were obtained (normal ranges are in brackets): Hb 9.0 (11.0–14.0 g/dL); mean corpuscular/cell volume (MCV) 58 (80–94 fl); mean corpuscular haemoglobin (MCH) 20 (24–31 pg); mean corpuscular haemoglobin count/concentration (MCHC) 28 (32–36 g/dL); platelets 260 (150–400 × 10^9/L); red blood cell count 5.5 (4–5 × 10^2). Which one of these is the MOST likely diagnosis?**

○ A Iron deficiency anaemia
○ B Sideroblastic anaemia
○ C Thalassaemia trait
○ D Lead poisoning
○ E Anaemia of chronic disorders

Extended Matching Questions

22. Theme: Blood and coagulation values

	Hb (g/dL)	Platelets (× 10⁹/L)	Total WCC (× 10⁹/L)	% Neutrophils	INR	(APTT) (sec)
A	10.5	42	10	30	1.10	30
B	12.2	340	6	50	1.02	33
C	6.0	40	15	60	1.15	31
D	7	20	2.0	5	1.10	35
E	18	150	18	60	1.3	52
F	10	190	5	5	0.99	32
G	10	28	15	60	2.5	74

APTT, activated partial thromboplastin time; INR, international normalized ratio; WCC, white cell count.

For each patient below select the appropriate haematological parameters listed above. Each option may be used once, more than once, or not at all.

○ 1. A 1-year-old girl with haemolytic uraemic syndrome.
○ 2. A 1-year-old boy with Wiskott–Aldrich syndrome.
○ 3. A normal 2-day-old newborn baby.

23. Theme: Bleeding disorders

	Platelets (× 10⁹/L)	INR	APTT (sec)	Factor VIII (μ/mL)	Factor IX (μ/mL)	Bleeding Time (min)	Fibrinogen (g/L)
Normal values (child)	140-400	0.6-1.17	28-40	0.5-1.09	0.36-136	< 10	1.5-3.8
A	280	0.9	48	0.3	0.6	12	2.1
B	262	1.0	60	0.9	0.1	7	2.7
C	250	1.0	30	0.7	0.8	15	3.0
D	6	1.05	30	0.9	0.9	12	3.3
E	340	0.99	55	0.001	1.0	6	2.8
F	50	2.8	76	0.4	0.2	Not done	0.5
G	310	1.5	50	1.0	0.5	Not done	3.2
H	150	2.7	62	1.0	0.2	Not done	2.8

For each patient below select the most appropriate set of laboratory values above. Each option may be used once, more than once, or not at all.

○ 1. An infant with Glanzmann's thrombasthenia.
○ 2. A neonate who is well, but who has constant bleeding from venepuncture sites and the umbilical stump.
○ 3. A 6-year-old boy with severe haemophilia A.

24. Theme: Associations with cancer in children

A   Beckwith–Wiedemann syndrome
B   Neurofibromatosis type I
C   Down syndrome
D   Ataxia telangiectasia
E   Xeroderma pigmentosum
F   Osgood–Schlatter disease
G   von Hippel–Lindau disease

For each of the patients below select a syndrome/disease from the above list that is closely associated with the diagnosis the patient suffers from. Each option may be used once, more than once, or not at all.

○   1. A 3-year-old girl with an optic glioma.
○   2. A 5-year-old boy with a Wilms tumour.
○   3. A 2-year-old girl with B cell non-Hodgkin's lymphoma.

25. Theme: Childhood malignancies

A   Hodgkin's disease
B   Wilms tumour
C   Neuroblastoma
D   Hepatoblastoma
E   Germ cell tumour
F   Osteogenic sarcoma
G   Acute lymphoblastic lymphoma

For each patient with the following oncological presentations, select the most appropriate causative malignancy from the above list. Each option may be used once, more than once, or not at all.

○   1. A 5-year-old boy with a 2-week history of a low-grade fever, signs of an upper respiratory infection, bilateral lower limb pain, cervical and inguinal lymphadenopathy, a mediastinal mass and petechiae. The blood count demonstrates pancytopenia.
○   2. A 13-year-old girl with a recent onset of a low-grade fever, painless bilateral cervical lymphadenopathy and a history of weight loss for the preceding 2–3 months.
○   3. A 2-year-old boy presenting with pallor, irritability, a limp, hypertension and a right-sided palpable abdominal mass.

answers

1. Iron deficiency anaemia

Answers: A D E

The most common cause of microcytic hypochromic anaemia in infancy is indeed iron deficiency. The prevalence of iron deficiency anaemia in inner cities in the UK ranges from between 10% and 30% of preschool children. Serum ferritin is a reliable indicator of total iron stores, rather than serum transferrin. A bone marrow aspiration, utilizing specific iron stains, is the gold standard for documenting total iron stores. Iron deficiency anaemia commonly presents from 6 months of age upwards in a term infant; this is due to the fact that at this stage maternally derived iron stores are becoming depleted. The ratio of the mean cell volume to the red cell count is extremely useful in differentiating iron deficiency anaemia from thalassaemia. In iron deficiency anaemia the ratio is generally less than 13 to 1 while in ~~more~~ thalassaemia it is greater than 13 to 1. Deficiencies in the immune system have been documented in iron-deficient children, especially T cell function and cell-mediated immunity.

[handwritten annotations: "more" and "less" in the margin]

2. Hereditary haemolytic anaemia

Answers: A D

Hereditary spherocytosis, an autosomal dominant condition, is the most common of the hereditary haemolytic anaemias seen in Northern Europe. Spherocytes are seen on the blood smear but the laboratory confirmation test is the osmotic fragility test and not the chromosome fragility test. G6PD is inherited in an X-linked recessive manner while pyruvate kinase deficiency is in an autosomal recessive manner. G6PD is confirmed by demonstrating inadequate levels of the G6PD enzyme activity in red cells. The Embden–Meyerhof pathway is associated with the metabolism of glucose to lactate. G6PD is an enzyme required to generate reducing power from glucose-6-phosphate in the hexose monophosphate shunt – an offshoot from the main Embden–Meyerhof pathway. Therefore in G6PD deficiency the Embden–Meyerhof pathway is intact while the hexose monophosphate shunt is not.

3. Aplastic anaemia

Answer: E

The majority of cases of aplastic anaemia are acquired rather then congenital. The majority of cases are idiopathic in origin. Despite the term aplastic anaemia, all three blood-lines can be affected in aplastic anaemia – resulting in anaemia, thrombocytopenia and leucopenia (specifically neutropenia). Erythropoietin is not effective treatment in aplastic anaemia. Bone marrow transplant is a well-recognised treatment modality – replacing the patient's pathological bone marrow with a compatible donor's bone marrow and thereby introducing normal haematopoietic stem cells that will proliferate. Autologous bone marrow transplantation (ablating the patient's bone marrow only to replace it again with their own previously harvested bone marrow stem cells) naturally plays no role.

4. Autoimmune haemolytic anaemia

Answers: A B C E

The direct antiglobulin test or direct Coombs test is positive in AIHA as this test detects antibody and complement on the red cell surface after sensitization has occurred. The most frequent cause of AIHA is due to an intercurrent viral infection. Spherocytes are characteristically seen on the blood smear. AIHA is divided into warm and cold types but this depends on the temperature at which the causative cell-bound antibody is best detected and not relative to the patient's temperature. The warm-type AIHA is associated with immunoglobulin G and is usually seen in multi-system disease whereas the cold-type AIHA is associated with IgM and is usually seen in infective causes. Multi-system disease-related AIHA, such as systemic lupus erythematosus (SLE), occurs predominantly in the adolescent.

5. ABO blood grouping system

Answers: D E

Children with blood group A will have the A antigen on the red cell membrane surface and will have anti-B antibodies. Children with blood group O have the O antigen (which does not produce an antigenic response) but they will possess anti-A and anti-B antibodies. These antibodies, produced against red cell membrane antigens, are called isohaemagglutinins and are not present at birth – indeed children less than 1 year of age will not reliably have isohaemagglutinins. These antibodies, or isohaemagglutinins, are present in immunocompetent older children and adults. Type O and type A blood groups collectively form over 80% of all the blood groups seen in the United Kingdom. The main aim of cross-matching a donor's blood with a recipient's blood is to ensure that the transfused blood does not contain red cells that the recipient's antibodies will react with.

6. Red cell physiology

Answers: C D E

The kidney, specifically the peritubular complex of the kidney, is the predominant site of erythropoietin production and not endothelial cells. Vitamin B_6 and not vitamin C is a coenzyme in the initial stage of haem synthesis. The mitochondria produce haem while ribosomes produce the globin chains. A molecule of haemoglobin is composed of four globin chains attached to their own haem moiety and the red cell does metabolize glucose only.

7. Leukocytes

Answers: A B E

Eosinophils do play a role in the body's defense against parasites by providing a histamine-mediated inflammatory response at the site of entry, thereby expelling the parasite. Mast cells are derived from basophils. A monocyte, rather than a neutrophil, is called a phagocyte once it has migrated into tissues from the blood stream. Neutrophils rather than lymphocytes contain myeloperoxidase – to aid in microbial killing. Band cells are immature neutrophils – the former and the latter collectively comprise the absolute neutrophil count.

8. von Willebrand disease

Answers: A C D

vWD is classified into at least three types (I, II and III). The most common, type I, accounts for at least 70% of patients with vWD and is due to a partial deficiency of von Willebrand factor (vWF). Type II, much less common, is due to an abnormally functioning vWF, and type III is due to a complete absence of vWF. Therefore the majority of vWD cases are due to a quantitative rather than a qualitative abnormality of vWF. The bleeding seen in vWD is characteristically mucous-membrane bleeding, excess bleeding from surgical or dental procedures, and easy bruising – but not characteristically in the form of petechiae. The platelet count is unaffected and the ristocetin co-factor activity will be decreased. Ristocetin, in the presence of vWF, causes platelet aggregation, therefore when vWF is deficient or when a qualitative defect of vWF exists, diminished aggregation of platelets will be seen. vWD is inherited in an autosomal dominant manner.

9. Neonatal alloimmune thrombocytopaenia (NAIT)

Answers: A C E

(NAIT) is a disorder caused by a fetomaternal platelet incompatibility analogous to that in Rhesus haemolytic disease, with maternal antiplatelet antibodies crossing the placenta and destroying fetal platelets. Antibodies directed against the human platelet-antigen-1a cause the majority of cases. The father has to be HPA positive while the mother has to be HPA negative for the same HPA for NAIT to occur. NAIT commonly occurs in the first-born child and does not require previous sensitization to have occurred. The platelet count is often severely reduced at birth rather than 5 days thereafter and treatment may include maternally donated platelets that are transfused into the fetus via the periumbilical route before birth.

10. Blood products

Answers: A B C E

Fresh frozen plasma (FFP) results from centrifuging out the cellular components of blood and therefore FFP will contain all of the coagulation factors and complement. Cryoprecipitate is collected following a controlled thaw of FFP and contains fibrinogen and factor VIII, as well as von Willebrand factor and factor XIII. As FFP and platelets may contain isohaemagglutinins, these two blood product transfusions should be ABO-compatible with the recipient. 1 unit of random donor platelets per 10 kg of patient bodyweight normally raises the platelet count in the region of 30–60 × 10⁹/L. The recommended volume for an FFP infusion is 10 ml/kg.

11. Coagulation

Answers: A B C E

It is true that all clotting factors are synthesized in the liver, while factor VIII is synthesized in both the liver and in the endothelium. Factor XIII deficiency does not prolong the INR nor the APTT. Factor XIII works by stabilizing the fibrin clot once fibrin has been formed and therefore does not interfere with the INR or the APTT. Factor XIII deficiency usually presents with prolonged bleeding from the umbilical stump once the necrotic umbilical cord has become dislodged, with recurrent intracranial bleeding, or with recurrent miscarriages. It is therefore prudent in patients presenting with recurrent intracranial bleeding who have a normal INR and APTT to go ahead and request specific factor XIII levels to rule out this potential rare deficiency. An isolated factor VII deficiency will elevate the INR only and not the APTT. An isolated factor II deficiency (prothrombin) results in a prolonged APTT, TT and INR.

12. Leukaemia in childhood

Answers: A B

Ninety-five per cent of all leukaemias in childhood are classified as acute; the remaining 5% are chronic myeloid leukaemia, while chronic lymphocytic leukaemia does not occur in childhood. Acute lymphoblastic leukaemia (ALL) accounts for approximately 80% of all acute leukaemias, the other 20% being acute myeloid leukaemia. ALL arises from an uncontrolled proliferation of clonal lymphoblasts. These lymphoblasts can either be of T cell or B cell origin, with the majority of ALL cases being of B cell origin. The cell of origin in acute myeloid leukaemia is a myeloblast, not a lymphoblast, and therefore definitely not of B cell origin.

13. Cancer in children

Answer: C

In the UK the incidence of childhood cancer is 1 in 600 and not 1 in 6000. Tumours of the brain and spinal cord are the most commonly occurring solid tumours, not neuroblastoma. Leukaemia accounts for 30–35% of all childhood malignancies while lymphoma is in the region of 10–15% therefore collectively they account for nearly 50% of all cases of childhood malignancies. The most common brain tumour is an astrocytoma, not a medulloblastoma, although the latter is the most common high-grade tumour in childhood. Boys are more affected than girls by childhood cancer, albeit slightly, with a ratio in the region of 1.3 to 1.

14. Prognostic signs in acute lymphoblastic leukaemia

Answers: A B D E

The presence of the Philadelphia chromosome confers an extremely poor prognosis and patients with this chromosome need intensive and aggressive chemotherapy. Patients outside the age range of 2–9 years carry a poor prognosis and, therefore, need more intensive treatment than patients within this age range. The presenting white cell count of greater than 50×10^9/L continues to be a poor prognostic sign, as does central nervous system disease, usually manifesting in the form of lymphoblasts within the cerebral spinal fluid.

15. Acute myeloid leukaemia

Answers: B D E

Treatment for AML is of much shorter duration than for acute lymphoblastic leukaemia (ALL) although it comprises far more intensive chemotherapy. Therapy normally lasts in the region of 6 months for AML treatment. Erythroblastic leukaemia is one of the sub-types of AML and has the designation of M6. AML is classified according to the FAB (French American British) classification system into eight sub-types (M0–M7): M0–M5 are assigned to the myeloid-differentiating cell, M6 to the erythrocyte-differentiating cell, and M7 to the platelet-differentiating cell. The most common sub-type of AML is not of B cell origin; this question is designed to confuse you with ALL where the cell of origin is either a B or T lymphoblast. The 5-year survival figures are now in the region of 50%. Secondary AML may result from previous chemotherapy used to treat other malignant conditions and it does carry an inferior prognosis relative to primary AML.

16. Tumour lysis syndrome

Answers: B D

ALL and B cell NHL are the pathologies most commonly giving rise to tumour lysis syndrome (TLS). AML may give rise to TLS but is not a common cause. TLS results from the intracellular contents of malignant cells being deposited into the circulation after cell lysis occurs, usually once treatment with chemotherapy has commenced – although in some cases TLS may occur prior to treatment even. Electrolyte imbalances – elevated phosphate, potassium and a decreased calcium level (due to precipitating out with the high

answers

phosphate) are commonly seen. Nuclear contents of the lysed cell give rise to increased uric acid (from the purine analogues of DNA). If the level reaches saturation point, uric acid crystals will precipitate out (as will phosphate crystals) eventually settling in the collecting system of the kidney, thus causing an obstructive uropathy and subsequent renal failure. Hyperhydration is the hallmark of effective treatment in preventing TLS in an attempt to flush the crystals out of the collecting system. Allopurinol, a xanthine oxidase inhibitor, decreases the production of uric acid, while urate oxidase (uricozyme) is the drug that increases the solubility of uric acid in order for it to be excreted in the urine and not crystallize out of solution.

17. Elevated α-fetoprotein (AFP)

Answer: All true

All the conditions in the question may cause an elevation of the α-fetoprotein level. The highest levels are usually seen in the malignant conditions such as hepatoblastoma, hepatocellular carcinoma (an uncommon malignancy in childhood) and a germ cell tumour comprising yolk sac elements. Regenerating liver tissue, such as seen in hepatitis for example, may cause an elevated AFP. Beckwith–Wiedemann syndrome is associated with a higher than normal AFP level in infancy and may be useful screening tool in this regard. Ataxia telangiectasia is associated with an elevated AFP and carcino-embryonic antigen (CEA).

18. Chemotherapeutic agents

Answer: All true

Vincristine is neurotoxic, manifesting predominantly as a peripheral neuropathy, ptosis or in severe cases vocal cord paralysis. The other reported side effects of vincristine are diminished reflexes, foot drop, abdominal pain, constipation and temporomandibular joint pain. Vincristine is given intravenously only and cannot be given intrathecally – with fatal consequences. Prednisone is a potent cytotoxic agent in that it potentially can induce remission when used alone in a patient suffering from leukaemia or lymphoma. Asparaginase asserts its action by depleting the body's store of asparagine, an essential amino acid. As a result the tumour cells cannot manufacture more protein and the cell eventually dies. Unfortunately, the production of other proteins within the body are affected as well, especially the coagulation proteins or clotting factors and anti-thrombin. Therefore, a patient may develop a clot or have a bleeding diathesis as a result of the asparaginase administration. Anthracyclines, of which daunomycin is one, are cardiotoxic. This normally manifests in the form of a cardiomyopathy, months to many years following administration. For this reason a patient receiving anthracycline treatment is followed regularly with an echocardiogram. Methotrexate is one of the drugs that can be administered via the oral, intravenous or intrathecal route.

19. Radiotherapy in children

Answer: All false

Craniospinal irradiation has the potential to cause growth hormone deficiency as well as causing decreased vertebral growth and therefore both the standing height and the sitting height of a child may be affected. Depending on the age of the child, an anaesthetic may be necessary to immobilize a young child for radiotherapy. Anaesthetic gases are not contraindicated in the radiotherapy suite. It is believed that the brain is nearly fully developed by the age of 7 years although cranial radiotherapy is not contraindicated in children under this age. The younger the child, the greater the devastating effects of radiotherapy will be and it is common clinical practice to attempt to avoid radiotherapy in children under 3 years of age if at all possible. The maximal tolerated dose of radiotherapy is a life-long dose and therefore it is not possible to safely irradiate an area that has already received the maximum radiation dose. Radiation-induced hypothyroidism and growth hormone deficiency are, unfortunately, permanent.

20. Chemotherapy-induced febrile neutropenic episodes

Answers: B C D

An absolute neutrophil count of $< 0.5 \times 10^9$/L is generally regarded as severe neutropenia, and a criterion used to define a febrile neutropenic episode. Temperatures above 38°C are generally regarded as febrile temperatures. It is true that a child who is neutropenic and who becomes febrile should be treated as a medical emergency as the potential for fulminant septicaemia is a distinct possibility. Patients should be seen immediately, a blood culture needs to be taken, and immediately thereafter broad spectrum intravenous antibiotics should be given. The general recommendation is that if the patient's fever persists for longer than 5 days it is prudent to investigate for an underlying fungal infection and to treat with an antifungal agent, usually with intravenous amphotericin. Paracetamol is contraindicated in the neutropenic child who is not on broad spectrum antibiotics as its antipyretic nature can mask an elevated temperature, thereby giving the patient, their family, and the medical team a false sense of security. Once the patient has been commenced on intravenous broad spectrum antibiotics, paracetamol may be used.

21. Thalassaemia trait

Answer: C

This question tests your ability to differentiate the potential causes of microcytic hypochromic anaemia. Iron deficiency anaemia will be the most common entity in this age group, followed by thalassaemia trait, and the final three causes (sideroblastic anaemia, lead poisoning, and anaemia of chronic disorders) will be way down the list. Therefore to distinguish between iron deficiency anaemia and thalassaemia trait, the history may be helpful. In this case if the dietary history is reliable, iron deficiency anaemia is possible, but not likely. The parents of this patient, being of Asian descent and distantly related, may be carriers of thalassaemia and therefore thalassaemia trait is a definite possibility. The platelet and red blood cell counts are two useful parameters in helping to distinguish iron deficiency anaemia from thalassaemia trait. The platelet count in iron deficiency anaemia is normally elevated, or is at least at the upper range of normal, while the red blood cell count is low. On the other hand the red blood cell count is normally elevated in thalassaemia trait while the haemoglobin is low, but not as low as that seen in iron deficiency anaemia. For the above reasons, the most likely diagnosis would be of thalassaemia trait.

22. BLOOD AND COAGULATION VALUES

1. C

Hb (g/dL)	Platelets ($\times 10^9$/L)	Total WCC ($\times 10^9$/L)	% Neutro-phils	INR	(APTT) (sec)
6.0	40	15	60	1.15	31

The haemolytic uraemic syndrome (HUS) occurs throughout the world and is the commonest cause of acute renal failure in children in North America and Western Europe. It is characterized by a haemolytic anaemia, thrombocytopenia and renal failure. The most common form occurs in children and is associated with a diarrhoeal illness. Item C has the most appropriate haematological parameters for the haemolytic uraemic syndrome in that there is anaemia and thrombocytopenia, with the other parameters being normal. One could confuse items C and D, but in D there is an associated neutropenia, which is generally not seen in the HUS syndrome.

2. A

Hb (g/dL)	Platelets ($\times 10^9$/L)	Total WCC ($\times 10^9$/L)	% Neutro-phils	INR	(APTT) (sec)
10.5	42	10	30	1.10	30

Wiskott–Aldrich syndrome, an X-linked recessive genetic condition, causes persistent thrombocytopenia and in its complete form also causes small platelets, atopy, cellular and humoral immunodeficiencies (particularly immunoglobulin deficiency, and an increased risk of autoimmune disease and haematological malignancies). Item A has the most appropriate haematological parameters for the Wiskott–Aldrich syndrome in that there is an isolated thrombocytopenia only.

3. E

Hb (g/dL)	Platelets ($\times 10^9$/L)	Total WCC ($\times 10^9$/L)	% Neutro-phils	INR	(APTT) (sec)
18	150	18	60	1.3	52

A normal 2-day-old neonate characteristically will have hematological parameters similar to item D in that the hemoglobin is slightly elevated, platelet count is normal, total white cell count is elevated relative to an older child and finally the INR and APTT are slightly prolonged.

23. BLEEDING DISORDERS

1. C

Platelets × 10⁹)	INR	APTT (sec)	Factor VIII (μ/mL)	Factor IX (μ/mL)	Bleeding Time (min)	Fibrinogen (g/L)
250	1.0	30	0.7	0.8	15	3.0

Glanzmann's thrombasthenia, caused by a deficiency of a protein (called glycoprotein IIb/IIIa) on the surface of the platelet, is a rare autosomal inherited (predominantly recessive but in some cases dominant) condition resulting in easy bruising and excessive bleeding after trauma or epistaxis. It is characterized by a normal platelet count but the platelets are functionally impaired due to the above glycoprotein deficiency and therefore do not aggregate. In patient C, the platelet count is normal but the bleeding time is prolonged – a characteristic of Glanzmann's thrombasthenia.

2. H

Platelets × 10⁹)	INR	APTT (sec)	Factor VIII (μ/mL)	Factor IX (μ/mL)	Bleeding Time (min)	Fibrinogen (g/L)
160	2.7	62	1.0	0.2	Not done	2.8

A well neonate with bleeding from venipuncture sites and the umbilical stump most likely has haemorrhagic disease of the newborn – in keeping with patient H's parameters: a prolonged INR and APTT together with a reduced factor IX level (a vitamin K-dependent factor) but with normal platelets.

3. E

Platelets × 10⁹)	INR	APTT (sec)	Factor VIII (μ/mL)	Factor IX (μ/mL)	Bleeding Time (min)	Fibrinogen (g/L)
340	0.99	55	0.001	1.0	6	2.8

Haemophilia A, an X-linked recessive bleeding disorder, due to a deficiency in factor VIII, is divided into three types depending on what percentage of normal factor VIII is present: mild (5–30%), moderate (1-5%) and severe (< 1% of normal). Patient E's parameters – a low factor VIII level together with a normal bleeding time – are in keeping with a patient with mild haemophilia A. This is not to be confused with patient A – where the factor VIII level is low but the bleeding time is prolonged – in keeping with von Willebrand disease. Haemophilia B (Christmas disease), a clinically similar condition, is not to be confused; here the factor IX level is reduced.

24. ASSOCIATIONS WITH CANCER IN CHILDREN

1.   B – Neurofibromatosis type I

Patients with neurofibromatosis type I are prone to develop central nervous system gliomas, particularly optic gliomas. These are low grade or benign tumours but due to their location can cause significant morbidity and potential mortality. The overgrowth syndromes, particularly Beckwith–Weidemann syndrome (macroglossia, organomegaly, omphalos and hemihypertrophy) are associated with Wilms' tumour and to a lesser extent hepatoblastoma as well.

2.   A – Beckwith–Weidemann syndrome

Wilms' tumour is associated with other syndromes, particularly WAGR syndrome (Wilms' tumour, aniridia, genitourinary abnormalities and mental retardation), Denys' Drash syndrome (pseudohermaphroditism, Wilms' tumour and nephrotic syndrome) and Perlman syndrome (phenotypically similar to Beckwith–Weidemann syndrome).

3.   D – Ataxia telangiectasia

Ataxia telangiectasia is a chromosomal breakage disorder affecting multiple symptoms that characteristically manifest primarily by ataxia, telangiectasia, and frequent sinopulmonary infections. It presents within the first 2 years of life, normally with ataxia. It is an autosomal recessively inherited disorder and both boys and girls are equally affected. Due to this condition being a chromosome breakage syndrome, there is an association with malignancy, particularly leukaemia and lymphoma.

25. CHILDHOOD MALIGNANCIES

1.   G – Acute lymphoblastic lymphoma

Acute lymphoblastic leukaemia (ALL) generally presents with signs and symptoms related to bone marrow failure, ie anaemia, thrombocytopenia, and secondary effects of leukopenia (infections). In addition, patients can present with extramedullary (outside the bone marrow) signs such lymphadenopathy, hepatomegaly, and splenomegaly. Bone pain, often presenting as a limp in the younger child, may be a presentation of presumed lymphoblast infiltration of the marrow cavity. The highest incidence of ALL occurs in patients aged 2–6 years.

2.   A – Hodgkin's disease

Hodgkin's disease, generally a disease of adolescents and young adults, is extremely uncommon under the age of 5 years. The most common presentation is that of painless cervical lymphadenopathy. The triad of symptoms, fever, night sweats and loss of weight are classified as B symptoms and occur in approximately 30–40% of patients, the frequency increasing with advanced stage of the disease.

3.   C – Neuroblastoma

The presenting symptoms of neuroblastoma are often non-specific and are, therefore, often overlooked as a potential aetiology in favour of more common paediatric conditions. It is a tumour that is derived from the sympathetic nervous system and therefore the primary site varies (adrenal 32%, rest of abdomen 28%, thorax 50%, pelvis 6%, neck 2% and other 16%). Presentation is often late and therefore metastatic disease, particularly to bone, is a common occurrence. This may lead to bone pain manifesting as irritability and/or a limp. Anaemia secondary to bone marrow infiltration is common. Catecholamines, produced by neuroblastoma cells, may result in metabolic effects, manifesting as hypertension, sweating and diarrhoea. The median age of onset is 2 years.

Immunology

Waseem Qasim

Multiple Choice Questions

1. Epstein–Barr virus
○ A is a member of the herpes virus family
○ B is usually associated with leukopenia
○ C can establish life-long latency
○ D causes haemolytic anaemia
○ E responds to intravenous ribavirin therapy

2. IgA deficiency
○ A is the commonest form of primary immunodeficiency
○ B usually presents as growth faltering
○ C has an association with coeliac disease
○ D is a contraindication to BCG (bacille Calmette–Guérin) immunisation
○ E increases the risk of transfusion reactions

3. Nitric oxide
○ A inhibits the aggregation of platelets
○ B is the active moiety of glycerol trinitrate
○ C production is inhibited by steroids
○ D dilates the arterial circulation
○ E increases pulmonary vascular resistance

4. Lyme disease
○ A may present with a larva migrans rash
○ B is best treated with cotrimoxazole in children
○ C is caused by a spirochaete
○ D causes cerebellar ataxia
○ E causes Guillain–Barré, syndrome

questions

5. Erythema nodosum is associated with

- ○ A sarcoidosis
- ○ B *Bartonella henselae* infection
- ○ C Crohn's disease
- ○ D ulcerative colitis
- ○ E streptococcal infection

6. The following are absolute contraindications to measles–mumps–rubella (MMR) vaccination

- ○ A autism
- ○ B attention deficit disorder
- ○ C HIV infection
- ○ D previous mumps infection
- ○ E hepatitis B infection

7. In Wiskott–Aldrich syndrome

- ○ A there are reduced numbers of large platelets
- ○ B psoriasis is common
- ○ C inheritance is X-linked
- ○ D immune cells have defective motility
- ○ E vasculitis is common

8. In haematopoietic stem cell transplantation

- ○ A umbilical cord blood may be used
- ○ B CD34 identifies stem cells
- ○ C the donor and recipient must have identical major histocompatibility complex (MHC) antigens
- ○ D donor T cells cause graft versus host disease
- ○ E growth retardation is a late complication

9. The polymerase chain reaction (PCR)

- ○ A requires monoclonal antibodies
- ○ B requires forward and reverse primers
- ○ C requires restriction digestion enzymes
- ○ D is used to quantify human immunodeficiency virus (HIV) load
- ○ E may be used to amplify RNA

10. Kawasaki disease is associated with

- ○ A hydrops of the gallbladder
- ○ B myocarditis
- ○ C erythema of BCG vaccination site
- ○ D desquamation of the perineum
- ○ E cranial nerve palsy

- **11. Members of the innate immune system include**
  - ○ A T lymphocytes
  - ○ B antimicrobial peptides
  - ○ C insulin-like growth factors
  - ○ D complement C3
  - ○ E lectins

12. Apoptosis
  - ○ A causes cellular shrinkage
  - ○ B is an inflammatory process
  - ○ C is mediated by caspases
  - ○ D is induced by tumour necrosis factor (TNF)
  - ○ E is induced by insulin

13. Disease-associated prions
  - ○ A replicate in red blood cells
  - ○ B resist proteinases
  - ○ C may be detected by polymerase chain reaction (PCR)
  - ○ D are inherited with mitochondria
  - ○ E accumulate in the tonsils

14. Following delivery, infants born to HIV-infected mothers should
  - ○ A receive high-dose cotrimoxazole
  - ○ B commence triple therapy
  - ○ C avoid breast feeding
  - ○ D be immunised with BCG
  - ○ E receive high-dose immunoglobulin

15. Recognised causes of thrombocytopenia are
  - ○ A phenytoin
  - ○ B carbamazepine
  - ○ C heparin
  - ○ D protamine sulphate
  - ○ E tranexamic acid

Best of Five Questions

16. **A 14-year-old boy undergoes a course of intensive chemotherapy. He is known to be seronegative for herpes zoster. He is visited by his sister, who develops chickenpox the next day. What would the MOST appropriate action be?**

○ A To start oral aciclovir immediately
○ B To start intravenous aciclovir immediately
○ C To administer zoster immune globulin within 48 hours
○ D To suspend his chemotherapy programme and observe
○ E To observe and administer zoster immune globulin if lesions develop

17. **Meningitis is suspected in a 3-week-old baby. Which of the following treatment combinations is MOST appropriate?**

○ A Vancomycin and cefotaxime
○ B Cefotaxime and aciclovir
○ C Ampicillin and cefotaxime
○ D Benzyl penicillin and gentamicin
○ E Vancomycin and gentamicin

18. **The MOST appropriate treatment for suspected scabies infestation in a 3-year-old child would be which of the following?**

○ A Benzyl benzoate
○ B Ketoconazole
○ C Permethrin
○ D Hydrocortisone
○ E Chlorhexidine

19. **Nontuberculous mycobacterial infection is suspected in a child with a single enlarged cervical lymph node. The MOST appropriate next step in management would be which of the following?**

○ A Fine needle biopsy of the node
○ B Complete surgical excision of the node
○ C Treatment with isoniazid for 3 months
○ D Treatment with rifampicin for 6 weeks
○ E Immunisation with BCG

20. **Osteomyelitis of the femur is suspected in a 4-year-old child. From the list below, which is the MOST likely organism to be involved?**

   ○ A Group B streptococcus
   ○ B *Salmonella*
   ○ C *Mycoplasma pneumoniae*
   ○ D *Staphylococcus aureus*
   ○ E *Haemophilus influenzae B*

21. **The sputum smear of the mother of a newborn is found to be positive for tuberculosis (TB). Congenital TB infection is excluded. The MOST appropriate action would be which of the following?**

   ○ A No further intervention
   ○ B X-ray radiography of the baby's chest in 2 weeks
   ○ C Immunise the baby with BCG
   ○ D Treat the baby with isoniazid
   ○ E Treat the baby with isoniazid, rifampicin and pyrazinamide

22. **Which of the following is the MOST effective treatment for chronic hepatitis C infection?**

   ○ A Interferon-α and ribavirin
   ○ B Ribavirin alone
   ○ C Interferon-α alone
   ○ D Lamivudine alone
   ○ E Interferon-α and lamivudine

Extended Matching Questions

23. Theme: Viral infections

A   Herpes simplex virus
B   Human herpes virus 6
C   Influenza virus
D   Adenovirus
E   Epstein–Barr virus
F   Cytomegalovirus
G   Hepatitis A
H   Hepatitis B
I   Measles
J   Mumps
K   Rubella

For each of the situations below, select the most likely causative agent from the list above. Each option may be used once, more than once, or not at all.

○   1. A 15-month-old infant presents to the emergency department with a 3-day history of high fevers without any localising signs. She suffers a short self-limiting febrile convulsion and is admitted for observation. The next day the fever lapses, but a red macular–papular rash develops over her trunk and abdomen.

○   2. A 10-year-old boy complains of headache and goes to bed early. The next morning he is found to be drowsy and confused. He is admitted to hospital where CT imaging reveals bilateral temporal lobe enhancement.

○   3. A 42-year-old man develops mild jaundice 1 month after a trip to Thailand. His 4-year-old son now presents with vomiting and diarrhoea. The child has been febrile and is thus receiving regular doses of paracetamol. His liver function tests are slightly deranged.

24. Theme: Techniques used in laboratory investigations

A   Southern blot
B   Northern blot
C   Western blot
D   Polymerase chain reaction (PCR)
E   Fluorescent in-situ hybridisation (FISH)
F   Enzyme-linked immunoassay (ELISA)
G   Flow cytometry

For each of the investigations below, select the most appropriate method of analysis from the list above. Each option may be used once, more than once, or not at all.

○   1. Detection of a 22q11 deletion on a sample of whole blood.
○   2. Detection of cytomegalovirus (CMV) in a sample of cerebrospinal fluid (CSF).
○   3. Measurement of CD4 : CD8 ratio in whole blood.

25. Theme: Childhood immunodeficiency

A   Chronic granulomatous disease
B   Chédiak-Higashi syndrome
C   Hyper-IgM syndrome
D   X-linked agammaglobulinaemia
E   Leukocyte adhesion deficiency (type 1)
F   Congenital neutropenia
G   Cyclical neutropenia

For the scenarios below, select the most likely diagnosis from the list above. Each option may be used once, more than once, or not at all.

1. A 3-year-old boy is investigated for recurrent deep skin infections. His mother reports that he had delayed separation of his umbilical cord and is under regular dental review for periodontitis. A surgical colleague examined an infected forearm site, and found there was little pus to drain and the procedure was complicated by delayed wound healing. His full blood count is as follows: haemoglobin (Hb) 12.2; white blood cells (WBC) 19.8; neutrophils 13.2; lymphocytes 6.0; platelets 456.

2. A diagnosis of sclerosing cholangitis is made in an 8-year-old boy who has been investigated for weight loss, abdominal pain and jaundice. He has a history of recurrent chest infections and diarrhoeal illness. One of his brothers had died of pneumonia at the age of 18 months.

3. A 13-year-old girl has severe cellulitis around the left eye. She has a history of similar infections and is troubled by recurrent bouts of mouth ulcers. Her mother also has a history of mouth ulcers and gingivitis.

answers

1. Epstein–Barr virus

Answers: A C D

Epstein–Barr virus (EBV) is a DNA virus. Like other members of the herpes family it may establish life-long latency (infection may re-activate in later life). Infection is usually associated with a leukocytosis, with atypical lymphocytes on the blood film. Serious complications of EBV infection include haemolytic anaemia, splenic rupture, myocarditis, encephalitis, and lymphoproliferative disease. There is no specific treatment of EBV. Steroids are often used to reduce airway swelling, or treat complications such as haemolytic anaemia. In immunocompromised patients ganciclovir may be of some benefit. Recently, rituximab (a monoclonal antibody against CD20) has been used to treat EBV-driven lymphoproliferative disease.

2. IgA deficiency

Answers: A C E

IgA deficiency is relatively common, affecting between 1 in 300 and 1 in 600 people. Most cases are subclinical in childhood, though they may present with atopy or recurrent infections of the respiratory tract or gastrointestinal system. There are known associations with autoimmune disorders, coeliac disease, Crohn's disease, ulcerative colitis and malignancies in older patients. Many patients will develop antibodies against immunoglobulin A (IgA), and are at increased risk of anaphylaxis following transfusions as the donated blood will harbour IgA.

3. Nitric oxide

Answers: A B C D

Nitric oxide (NO) can be derived from endothelial cells, neuronal cells and macrophages. It inhibits the aggregation of white cells and platelets. Steroids inhibit macrophage nitric oxide synthases and reduce NO production. The main source of NO is the vascular endothelium, which is continuously dilated by basal synthesis of NO. Pulmonary vascular resistance is reduced by NO, and hence the gas may be used in patients who are difficult to ventilate. It is the active moiety of nitro-vasodilators, including glyceryl trinitrate.

4. Lyme disease

Answers: C D E

Lyme disease is caused by the spirochaete *Borrelia burgdorferi*, and is transmitted by ticks carried by wild deer and other animals. The characteristic rash is called erythema migrans, and evolves around a central bite up to 21 days after exposure. Most cases respond to a 3-week course of Amoxil or erythromycin. Complications include arthritis, cardiac involvement, and hepatitis. Neurological complications include cranial nerve palsies, Guillain–Barré syndrome, cerebellar ataxia and aseptic meningitis. Diagnosis is usually based on history and clinical findings, with supportive serology for *Borrelia*.

5. Erythema nodosum

Answer: All true

Erythema nodosum describes red or dark raised ovoid lesions of 1–3 cm on the shin, usually in girls over the age of 6 years. Systemic causes include sarcoidosis, Crohn's disease, ulcerative colitis and vasculitis. Infective causes include *Streptococcus* infection, mycoplasma, tuberculosis, cat scratch disease (*Bartonella henselae*), Epstein–Barr virus, and histoplasmosis. Sulfonamides and the contraceptive pill can also cause this reaction.

6. MMR vaccination

Answer: All false

MMR is a live vaccine, and is contraindicated in patients with significant immunodeficiency, including those who have been on steroids during the previous 3 months, or those undergoing chemotherapy during the previous 6 months. The vaccine should be delayed if the child is febrile, or has another live vaccination in the previous 3 weeks. It should not be given during pregnancy. In the UK, it is recommended that children with HIV should not receive BCG, or vaccines for yellow fever or oral typhoid. However, they should be given routine inactivated vaccines and inactivated polio immunisation. MMR may be given as long as the child is not severely immunosuppressed at the time. Autism and attention deficit disorders are not contraindications to MMR, nor is there any evidence that MMR causes autism.

7. Wiskott–Aldrich syndrome

Answers: C D E

Wiskott–Aldrich syndrome (WAS) is X-linked. There is classically a triad of thromobocytopenia, eczema, and immunodeficiency. Platelets are small and have reduced volume. Associated features include vasculitis and autoimmunity, and a predisposition to lymphoproliferative diseases in later life. The underlying defect is due to loss of the WAS protein, which is important for cytoskeletal organisation and cell motility. The disease can be cured by bone marrow transplantation, and this should ideally be undertaken in children aged less than 5 years if a fully matched donor is available.

8. Haematopoietic stem cell transplantation

Answers: A B D E

Haematopoietic stem cells (HSC) may be derived from bone marrow harvests or leukopheresis after a course of granulocyte-colony stimulating factor (GCSF). Umbilical cord blood collected at the time of delivery is a rich source of HSC and cord blood banks are being established. CD34 is a cell surface molecule that is routinely used to identify and select HSC. Patients may have a fully MHC-matched sibling donor, or there may be an unrelated matched volunteer donor. The risk of graft versus host disease (GVHD) is greatly increased if mismatched donors are used, although on occasion parental haplo-identical donors have to be used. GVHD is mediated by donor T cells, and T cells can be removed from the graft to reduce the risk. Late complications of HSCT include impaired immune reconstitution, growth retardation, autoimmunity and endocrine dysfunction.

9. Polymerase chain reaction

Answers: B D E

In polymerase chain reaction (PCR) reactions, two oligonucleotide primers (15–30 base pairs in size) are mixed with the target DNA, a mixture of deoxyribonucleoside triphosphates (dNTPs) and thermostable Taq polymerase. Primers are designated forward and reverse, depending on which strand of DNA they bind. There are three stages to each PCR cycle:

- Heating to 95°C causes the DNA strands to separate (denaturation)
- Cooling to 54°C allows the primers to anneal to each strand
- Heating to 72°C results in incorporation of dNTPs.

The process results in exponential expansion of DNA after each cycle. Target RNA may be amplified by using reverse transcriptase (RT) to convert it to template DNA before use in a PCR reaction. HIV is an RNA virus that can be detected and quantified using an RT-PCR reaction. This is now routinely used to follow the efficacy of anti-retroviral treatment on HIV load.

10. Kawasaki disease

Answer: All true

The established criteria for the diagnosis of Kawasaki disease are 5 days of fever plus four of the following:

- cervical lymphadenopathy
- non suppurative conjunctivitis
- exanthem
- swelling or desquamation of the hands or feet
- oropharyngeal inflammation.

Additional features include irritability, meningitis, iridocyclitis and arthritis. Dilatation or hydrops of the gallbladder is recognised. Erythema of a BCG immunisation site is a characteristic feature. Peripheral and cranial nerve palsies may occur. The development of coronary arteritis may lead to aneurysms and thrombosis, though all parts of the heart may be involved.

11. Innate immune system

Answers: B D

The innate or non-specific immune system is the first line of defence against pathogens. It has many components, including mechanical barriers (skin, mucous secretions) and soluble factors (complement, mannose-binding lectin) as well as neutrophils and macrophages. Anti-microbial peptides, such as β-defensins are proteins secreted by endothelial cells. Specific immunity is provided by T cells and B cells, and results in the generation of immune memory, resulting in rapid responses on subsequent challenge by a given pathogen.

12. Apoptosis

Answers: A C D

Apoptosis results in programmed cell death and is non-inflammatory. Apoptosis is needed for embryonic development in utero and tissue homeostasis in adult life. Apoptosis may be induced by soluble factors such as TNF-binding death receptors or the withdrawal of growth factors (eg insulin-like growth factors). During apoptosis cells shrink, chromatin condenses, with endonuclease activation and DNA cleavage. Caspases are important mediators of apoptotic signals within cells. Mutations in some genes or over-expression of others (eg *bcl-2*) may lead to a failure of apoptosis and the formation of tumourogenic cell populations.

13. Disease-associated prions

Answers: B E

According to the prion hypothesis, disease-causing prions are corrupted versions of naturally occurring prion proteins found on cell surfaces. Once corrupted they resist proteinase degradation, are heat stable, and are insensitive to ultraviolet light damage. Prions cause transmissible spongiform encephalopathies (TSEs) such as BSE in cattle and Creutzfeldt–Jacob disease (CJD) in man. In 1996, new-variant CJD was first described and is thought to be caused by bovine prions entering the human food chain. Such prions are detectable in tonsil tissue. They do not encode genetic material and thus are not detectable by PCR.

14. Infants born to HIV-infected mothers

Answer: C

In the UK, the current guidelines recommend treatment of infants of HIV-positive mothers with zidovudine (AZT) from birth. Nelfinavir is an alternative agent that may be used, in particular if the mother is known to have

answers

developed resistance to AZT. Triple therapy is not usually indicated at birth, but may be initiated if there were a rising viral load or a falling CD4 count. PCR for HIV is usually performed within 48 hours, and repeated at 6 weeks. If both are negative, therapy can be stopped and the baby followed up until antibody negative. Babies should not be breast fed, and should not receive BCG vaccination. Cotrimoxazole would usually be given from 6 weeks of age. There is no indication for immunoglobulin therapy.

15. Thrombocytopenia

Answers: A B C

Drug-induced thrombocytopenia may be as a result of direct toxicity on the megakaryocytes or as a result of immune-mediated platelet consumption. Common causes in children include phenytoin, carbamazepine, chloramphenicol, and co-trimoxazole. Heparin may induce immune-mediated platelet elimination 7–10 days after starting treatment. Protamine sulphate is used to reverse heparin anticoagulation effects and tranexamic acid is a pro-coagulant.

16. C – Administer zoster immune globulin within 48 hours

Chickenpox is infectious 24–48 hours before the rash appears, until the final lesion has crusted. In an immunodeficient patient who is not immune to varicella zoster there is a clear indication for zoster immune globulin (ZIG). There would be a case for aciclovir to be given 7 days after exposure (minimum incubation time), but it is of little benefit until lesions develop. It may be necessary to suspend the programme of chemotherapy, but the most appropriate action is to give ZIG within 48 hours.

17. C – Ampicillin and cefotaxime

Under the age of 4 weeks, the common causes of meningitis include: group B streptococci; *Escherichia coli*; *Listeria monocytogenes*. Other pathogens such as *Haemophilus influenzae*, *Staphylococcus*, and *Klebsiella* spp are less frequent. From the list of answers, the most appropriate presumptive therapy would be with cefotaxime and ampicillin. Cefotaxime provides broad spectrum cover against streptococci and Gram-negative organisms and the inclusion of ampicillin is essential to cover *Listeria* infections.

18. C – Permethrin

The immune response to the mite *Sarcoptes scabiei humanis* causes itchy skin eruptions, often with an eczematous rash and excoriations. There may be burrows on the palms, soles and digits. The mite can survive for up to 36 hours away from the human host. All family members should be treated, and clothing and bed-linen should be washed. Treatment should be with permethrin (Lyclear) or malathion (Derbac) lotions. Older preparations, such as benzyl benzoate, should be avoided in children. Ketoconazole is an antifungal agent and is not indicated. There may be an indication for systemic antibiotics if lesions become infected.

19. B – Complete surgical excision of the node

Incomplete excision or needle biopsy may lead to chronic drainage from the site. The preferred treatment for nontuberculous lymphadenopathy is complete surgical excision while the node is firm and encapsulated. Usually, no further treatment is required. Anti-tuberculous medication is required for 3–6 months if incomplete excision is suspected, or if there is dissemination. This should be guided by culture and sensitivity data, but a combination of two drugs (from ciprofloxacin, clarithromycin, rifampicin or rifabutin) should be used. If tuberculous infection cannot be excluded, treatment with rifampicin, isoniazid and pyrazinamide should be given.

20. D – *Staphylococcus aureus*

Osteomyelitis 3–10 years is more common in boys than in girls and there may be a history of trauma. The most commonly involved organism is *Staphylococcus aureus* and treatment should be intravenous flucloxacillin (plus fusidic acid). Other causes are *Streptococcus pneumoniae* or possibly *Escherichia coli*. In infants under 2 years of age alternative organisms include Group B streptococcus and *Haemophilus influenzae* type B. In patients with sickle cell disease, *Salmonella* and Gram-negative infections should be considered. Treatment may require surgical debridement and antibiotics should be given for 6 weeks.

21. D – Treat the baby with isoniazid

Congenital TB has been excluded but as the mother is smear positive then the neonate is at high risk and should be separated from the mother. The mother is considered infectious until she has completed the first 2 weeks of combination therapy with three or four drugs. The neonate should receive 3 months of isoniazid (and pyridoxine supplements) and should then be re-assessed for TB with chest X-ray, gastric aspirates, and tuberculin skin test. If all is well at this time then BCG should be given and isoniazid stopped.

22. A – Interferon-α and ribavirin

A combination of interferon-α and ribavirin has been shown to be effective in chronic hepatitis C infection, and is given for 6–12 months. Treatment is usually initiated on the basis of changes in liver biopsy histology, and success is tracked by measuring viral loads. Interferon-α alone is less effective and ribavirin used alone is ineffective. Lamivudine is used in hepatitis B infection. Interferon-α is of benefit in chronic granulomatous disease and in treating atypical mycobacterial infection in patients with defects of the interleukin-12/interferon-α axis.

23. VIRAL INFECTIONS

1.   B – Human herpes virus 6 (HHV-6)

HHV-6 is thought to infect 90% of infants by 2 years of age. The pattern of high fevers for 3 days without an obvious cause is characteristic. Febrile seizures are a relatively common mode of presentation. The roseola rash often appears as fever subsides, and may be macular or macular–papular and usually begins centrally, spreading later to the limbs and resolving in 48–72 hours. Although other viruses such as measles may cause a similar rash, the timing and fever pattern favour HHV-6.

2.   A – Herpes simplex virus

Though most of the viruses listed may cause meningoencephalitis, temporal lobe involvement is characteristic of herpes simplex virus infection. Cerebrospinal fluid (CSF) examination usually reveals a raised cell count, often with red cells present, and raised protein, but normal glucose level. The presence of the virus may be confirmed using PCR detection techniques. Treatment would be with high-dose intravenous aciclovir for 21 days.

3.   G – Hepatitis A

In early childhood hepatitis A usually causes self-limiting diarrhoea and vomiting. Mild hepatitis is common, though children rarely develop jaundice. There is often a nursery or home contact who has passed on the virus through the faecal–oral route. In this case it seems to have been the father. Though hepatitis B is prevalent in the far east, it is only transmitted by the blood borne route and does not cause diarrhoea.

24.   LABORATORY TECHNIQUES

1.   E – Fluorescent in-situ hybridisation (FISH)

FISH makes use of fluorescent-labelled probes to detect monosomies, trisomies, chromosomal deletions and translocations. Lymphocytes isolated from whole blood can be activated to divide and analysed in metaphase using FISH.

2.   D – Polymerase chain reaction (PCR)

PCR is very useful for the detection of small amounts of viral DNA, and is routinely used to detect CMV in CSF.

3.   G – Flow cytometry

Flow cytometry uses specific antibodies against cell surface molecules (and intracellular proteins) linked to excitable marker molecules. The technique is routinely used to identify T cell subsets based on CD4 and CD8 expression.

25. CHILDHOOD IMMUNODEFICIENCY

1.   E – Leukocyte adhesion deficiency (type 1)

The history is characteristic of an underlying defect of neutrophils. The neutrophil count is raised, thereby excluding congenital neutropenia, and making cyclical neutropenia unlikely. Chronic granulomatous disease may present in this manner (and a nitroblue tetrazolium (NBT) test should be performed to exclude it) but one would expect pus at the site of infections. The history of delayed cord separation and delayed wound healing is strongly suggestive of leukocyte adhesion deficiency type 1. This is a defect of the CD18 molecule on neutrophils and lymphocytes which leads to impaired cell migration. Thus, there is usually a persistent neutrophilia, but as cells are unable to target migration to sites of infection, very little pus formation occurs.

2.   C – Hyper-IgM syndrome

The scenario suggests X-linked immunodeficiency and the history of sclerosing cholangitis points towards hyper-IgM syndrome. This is an X-linked disorder of the CD40 ligand, an important T cell costimulatory molecule. Affected boys are predisposed to infections from early infancy, and are particularly susceptible to *Cryptosporidium* infections. This may lead to abdominal pain and severe diarrhoea, and may be associated with sclerosing cholangitis.

3.   G – Cyclical neutropenia

Cyclical neutropenia is an autosomal dominant disorder of haematopoicsis, in which patients become neutropenic for 3–6 days on a regular cycle of 3–4-weeks. The disorder is associated with mutations of the neutrophil elastase gene (*ELA2*) but it is not known why bone-marrow production of neutrophils is cyclical.

Index

This index covers Volume I and Volume II. The volumes are indicated by roman numerals, I and II.

index

index

index

index

index

index

index

index